Waterbirth

An attitude to care

To my father
who was my shining light
in both my personal
and professional lives

Waterbirth
An attitude to care

Second edition

Dianne Garland SRN, RM ADM, PGCEA, MSc

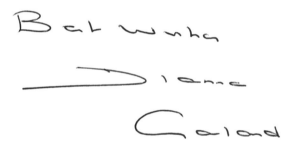

Best wishes
Diane
Galand

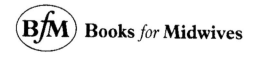
BfM **Books** *for* **Midwives**

OXFORD AUCKLAND BOSTON JOHANNESBURG MELBOURNE NEW DELHI

Books for Midwives
An imprint of Butterworth-Heinemann
Linacre House, Jordan Hill, Oxford OX2 8DP
225 Wildwood Avenue, Woburn, MA 01801-2041
A division of Reed Educational and Professional Publishing Ltd

℞ A member of the Reed Elsevier plc group

First published 1995
Second edition 2000

British Library Cataloguing in Publication Data
A catalogue record for this book is available from the British Library

ISBN 0 7506 5202 0

Printed and Bound in Great Britain by MPG, Bodmin, Cornwall

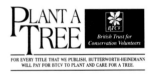

Contents

Acknowledgements

I would like to express my gratitude to the families and staff at Maidstone Hospital.

Introduction

Welcome to a guide on using water in midwifery practice, written by a midwife who has used hydrotherapy in her work for the past twelve years. The book will explore the practical issues of setting up a service and the implications for practice in the light of recent events. It also explores issues related to professional accountability and responsibility, particularly in the light of the controversy surrounding the legal responsibility of midwives providing this type of care. I have drawn on my personal experiences and visits to water birthing centres in America and Europe, and papers presented at ICM (International Confederation of Midwives) 1996 and 1999, sharing with you the care and practice of water labour/birth in a variety of settings. Many units have problems with setting up a water birthing facility and I have utilised my experiences at Maidstone over the past twelve years to assist the reader in the practical aspects and educational requirements.

Chapters are included on the issues of maternal and newborn physiology and practical aspects of care. The last three chapters review research that is currently being undertaken and ways of tackling areas of concern, with a chapter entitled 'What If...?'. Appendices cover the topics of maternal hyperthermia and neonatal interdependency on the mother, supporting parents at home waterbirths and setting up waterbirth parentcraft sessions.

Although written by one author, the last chapter includes accounts from other health professionals and parents' stories.

This book should act as a starting point, a foundation on which to build, or develop, a service that is sensitive and proactive to change.

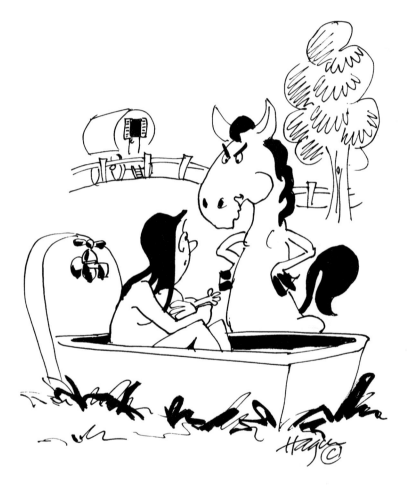

CHAPTER ONE

Midwives' accountability and responsibility

This chapter addresses the issues surrounding midwifery accountability and litigation in today's society. All the areas interlink, since we cannot practice as autonomous midwives without being aware of, and involved in, supervision and accountability.

Professional accountability

I would like to tackle three areas from the Code of Professional Conduct, 1984, which was issued following the formation of the United Kingdom Central Council (UKCC) in 1979 (UKCC, 1984 and UKCC, 1998). The areas are professional knowledge and competence, knowing your limitations and working together.

Professional knowledge and competence

3. *Take every reasonable opportunity to maintain and improve professional knowledge and competence.*

We all know that midwifery practice only really develops once we qualify. As midwives, refresher courses and continuing education are part and parcel of our work. So what happens with regard to using water in our practice? Part of this is based on how we view water labours/births. Is it an adaptation of normal midwifery practice or an area of extended limits of practice?

It is therefore imperative that all opportunities are utilised to enhance existing knowledge or develop new learning experiences. What learning has been offered regarding waterbirth? It may be appropriate to attend 'water' sessions, where clinical and practical issues are discussed. Many such sessions and workshops are available around the country and shared learning also occurs worldwide. In line with PREP these educational sessions should be recorded in your professional profile.

Education should be a lifelong process and even though I have been undertaking waterbirths for many years I am continually amazed at how much I still have to learn.

In what other ways can we learn and maintain skills? It should be possible to have access to videos and articles on waterbirths in a central, accessible area. Is this information regularly updated and reviewed in the light of current knowledge?

Some midwives have sought out clinical opportunities and have visited waterbirthing units, and skill-shared with colleagues with a greater degree of experience.

Whilst I believe it is the responsibility of each individual midwife to fulfil this section of the code, I also believe that supervisors of midwives should make every effort to be aware of resources available locally.

Knowing your limitations

4. Acknowledge any limitations of competence and refuse in such cases to accept delegated functions without first having received instruction with regard to those functions and having been assessed as competent.

This is often seen as a difficult issue, since in practice settings midwives may feel that identifying limitations could be seen as a failing. Indeed this has been indicated to me as both a midwife and a supervisor. On the contrary, I would see this recognition of need as positive and not negative. It takes a great deal of strength by an individual midwife to admit that she feels unable or unwilling to perform waterbirths.

What support is given by managers and supervisors may be dependent on their own viewpoint and experience. Having identified a limitation in skill, learning opportunities should be directed to the midwife who should be supported until she feels confident and competent to take on that skill – however long that takes. I do not believe unrealistic expectations and demands should be placed upon midwives; we all have our own particular skills and knowledge to offer the families in our care.

Working together

5. Work in a collaborative and cooperative manner with other healthcare professionals and recognise and respect their particular contributions within the healthcare team.

It is regrettable that the teamwork aspect of the Code must be mentioned, but though we all work in health services, whether in the private or public sector, it is sometimes lost. Teamwork is fundamental to providing high standards for the clients within our care. We may all have separate objectives for our day-to-day work, but whatever our own objectives the common goal of service provision is paramount.

In the current health service the client may almost be lost in the drive for efficiency, effectiveness and economy. The major changes to the UK health service have leant towards improved standards, choice in caregiver and place of service provision. In reality this may be occurring when each group of professionals is striving to protect their own 'hidden agenda'. In these difficult times of cost savings and efficiency, it is vital that professionalism, teamwork and mutual respect do not get buried.

It is well recognised that midwives are in a very different situation than nurses. We have a separate *Code of Practice* (UKCC, 1998) and *Midwives Rules* (UKCC, 1998) and, although issued by the UKCC, they are seen as complementary to, and not separate from, nursing codes. The midwifery profession fought hard to maintain a separate identity when *Project 2000* was introduced. Education was seen as fundamental to maintaining a distinct profession, with its own accountability and responsibility.

Developing new skills

Midwives rules and code of practice 1998:

> *Developments in midwifery care can become an integral part of the role of the midwife and are then incorporated in the initial preparation of the midwife. You must make sure that you become competent in such new skills...*

For midwives, the incorporation of water labours/births into initial practice may be related to the local clinical and educational institutions' access to specialists with this knowledge. It is vital that we take advantage of all local, national and international presentations regarding waterbirths. Much is written about waterbirths, both in the professional and consumer press, and this should be readily available to midwives in a central locality. The topic of midwives' education will be expanded upon in further chapters.

Radical changes are currently taking place within our sphere of practice, as we work in partnership with other health professionals to ensure that families receive the highest standards of care. This unique partnership is nothing new, but the power base is now shifting, with the midwife's role as facilitator, empowering women to regain control over their pregnancies and delivery.

The role of midwifery supervision

Supervision of Midwives was written into *The Midwives Act 1902* and despite several later Acts (1936, 1951 and 1974) this statutory obligation has basically remained unchanged. It is still required of supervisors to maintain identified set objectives. These are as follows:

- standard setting
- ensuring competent practitioners
- support to staff who are having difficulties
- identification of continuing training needs
- protection of the public.

  (Cited Jenkins and Murphy, 1993, pp.31-39)

At the present time midwifery is the only 'caring' profession that has this type of regulation, although other disciplines are reviewing this type of support. In its true form supervision should be there to facilitate practice and maintain standards, and also to protect the public. Unfortunately what has happened is that supervision has been inherently linked with the manager's role. Indeed many managers are supervisors and have this role written into their job descriptions. This situation is now being addressed in many units, where clinical grade midwives and educationalists are being appointed as supervisors. Not only does it provide a direct clinical link between supervision and practice, but it opens other avenues of debate and support as educationalists become involved in supervision. This can only benefit and strengthen the role of midwifery supervision.

Whether this is appropriate, when we look at the objectives above, is outside the scope of this book. It is, however, apparent to me that irrespective of who is supervisor, manager, tutor or clinician, they should provide an environment for practice that is supportive for change. Supervisors will also need to be available in such a way to provide 'a means of providing care for the carers' (Barber, 1994, pp.15-25).

Professional communication systems

One issue that should be addressed early on is communication. As discussed later in this book, holding joint discussions and involving all those who may have a vested interest pays dividends later. Information must be available to all clients regardless of social or ethnic background. Studies cited by Kirkham in Midwifery Practice: A Research Based Approach (Alexander *et al*, 1993) record the immense differences between the information given and received by different groups. It is vital, therefore, that water labour/birth advice is accessible to midwives in an easy to read format.

Avenues for communication may include parentcraft classes, written information and possibly personal interviews depending on circumstances. In my experience a combination of all three assists in setting the goal posts that over the past years have reduced areas of conflict or confrontation.

AIMS (1996) and the NCT (1995) are two booklets on waterbirth that should be made available to women in our care. Separate parentcraft sessions have been running at Maidstone for many years and these have been well received and evaluated. See Appendix III for details.

Inherent within this communication system is the fact that we assume that clients have expectations which they can articulate to their caregivers. Is it appropriate for individual midwives to give all the information required by parents and colleagues, or should a midwife who has a special interest in providing this educational service be identified? The fundamental point here is that all parents receive up-to-date and unbiased information that is related to the current knowledge base of midwifery.

Litigation and waterbirth

One cannot work within today's midwifery practice without being aware of the risk of litigation. I believe this is not a new situation but over the past few years this issue has become higher profile, and of course, changes to the legal aid system have assisted more parents in claiming damages against professionals (Mason and Edwards, 1993).

The issue of client choice versus legal implications has been discussed widely over the last few years. In Street (1997) the whole scenario of women's choice versus the midwife's legal position is described, together with the place of the legal status of the fetus as an added element in this complex situaton. It is vital that local guidelines are written. These should be agreed by all staff involved in care (including paediatricians, obstetricians and midwives) and shared with the parents in an open supportive environment. These guidelines need to be regularly evaluated (having already been based on current evidence) and altered in the light of changes to practice or new evidence.

Another issue is vicarious liability, which most midwives have received through their employer since the introduction of the NHS in 1948. This situation is radically altering as more midwives set up in independent practice, or work in other fields outside their normal NHS contract. I have highlighted this issue in Chapter Six on aquanatal swimming.

There can be little doubt that the number of cases of litigation have steadily increased over the past years but cases against midwives have, thankfully, remained few. One should also view this increase in the light of the general increase in obstetrical interventions and society's attitudes at the present time. Recent adverse publicity on the rising tide of caesarean sections is a prime example.

Recommendations for practice

- Dingwall cited by Alexander, Levy and Roch (1993) writes:

  The legal process can [also] be a cruel exposure of failures in teamwork. If one professional group has adopted policies and practices at odds with those of the others, a plaintiff's lawyer will have a field day with the discrepancies. In effect, though, the objective of the tort system is to encourage good practice, so that if your practice is soundly based, the result should not be a penalty for your employer.

- Records should be kept as contemporaneously as possible (Rule 42, *Midwives Rules* 1993).

- Is practice based on clearly stated policies and guidelines based on up to date knowledge and research? Are these policies communicated to all staff?
- Do you receive regular teaching, review and audit meetings?

Midwifery practice and politics

Midwifery practice may well have been embodied in statute, but whether this has protected us could be seen in the wider arena of political control. Professionalism is based on several markers, as identified by Downe and Kirkham (1993):

> *Constituting a profession... factors such as control over the parameters of work, self regulation and the existence of a unique body of knowledge are taken into account... society must feel a need for such an occupation's skills and the profession in turn, will have a considerable effect upon the prevailing social perception of its activities.*

A typical scenario of the last part of this quote is the recent advertising campaign for an airway company. In their television commercial a pregnant woman delivers, prematurely, on board the plane with, apparently, little assistance from two stewardesses. The concept here may be to visualise the skills of the airline, but it does little to show midwifery as a highly skilled profession. On a similar point, the TV series 'Men Behaving Badly' portrayed two young men as homebirth tub hirers! Despite the fact that the tub burst during use, waterbirth was shown as part of a comical scenario. Such instances can only add fuel to the fire that waterbirth is 'trendy' rather than 'normal' midwifery practice. This may seem pedantic but if we are to maintain our position in society, then it is vital that we are seen within the unique context of a profession.

Set within this scene is the control issue of who steers maternity care forward. A power struggle is ensuing in some areas between obstetricians, midwives and general practitioners. If you include those new NHS managers who may not be from the same professional groups, it is easy to see why conflict could occur. This is not only disagreeable for the professionals involved but for the mothers who often find themselves in the middle of this situation.

I am happy to state that this is not my experience. I have always received

support from colleagues in both the 'caring' professions and administration managers. Communicating with all those who may be involved
pays dividends and interprofessional rivalry has not occurred. Indeed a
partnership for care has developed and I believe this is partly why in my
clinical experience difficulties have not developed.

Conclusion

Tremendous changes are occurring within midwifery and it is a unique
opportunity to regain the professional standing that midwives once had.
Independent midwives, team and caseload management will offer women
choice in care and in partnership with other professionals, they will be
able to choose their care giver. Change never comes easily and I believe
that part of the problems that have been experienced elsewhere may be
due to the political and social arena within which we are working.

CHAPTER TWO

Pioneering hydrotherapists

Water has long been known for its therapeutic value – ancient rituals and traditions have developed surrounding water. Whilst not all has been substantiated with true evidence, a greater awareness of its value has been made available through the writings of Odent (1990). A strong spiritualistic and mystic link may well exist between humans and water, this being one reason why we are so drawn to water in life. In *We are all Water Babies*, Odent (1994) explores this connection to water by looking at the relationship we, as land mammals, have with sea mammals, particularly dolphins. In the book Odent delves deeply into the ability of newborns to 'swim' in water. The amazing photographs taken by co-author Jessica Johnson allow us the opportunity to see the world of newborns in water. During the journey through the book, we share with Odent and Johnson the relaxing effects of water on both mother and fetus.

Odent states:

> *The relaxing effects of water are transmitted to the fetus, whether the mother is submerged in it or simply nearby.*

I would suggest that this book makes wonderful background reading for anyone wishing to explore the use of water in today's maternity practice.

Anyone who has visited Niagara or Victoria Falls cannot fail to be inspired by their beauty and power. Each year thousands of people travel to these destinations to stand and admire their strength. Water has always played a vital part in our society. Long ago our major settlements were sited on rivers and the ocean. The potential value and strength of waterways established the great sea trading nations of the world. Britain was one such nation and even before 'Britannia ruled the waves' trading nations existed in the Far East. Even today the oceans provide lifelines and great canals have been built and fought over in a bid to control 'water'. The Panama and Suez canals are prime examples of man's attempts to control the power that goes with speeding up seafaring nations' trading opportunities.

In today's changing environment, one of our major concerns is the earth's resources and the continuing pollution of the world's oceans. We are told of over-harvesting fish stocks – it seems to be in the news almost weekly. Without controls these stocks could become decimated. Our newspapers and television screens have, over the past few years, shown us the horrors of chemical and oil pollution occurring at sea. Shipping disasters appear all too often. In Alaska, Spain and Shetland we have been confronted by oil spills that have wreaked havoc on local wildlife. Some instances have not even been due to 'human error' but due to man's self-destructive attitude and disregard for his environment. The full impact will probably not be fully obvious until the next century. Water can, therefore, be seen to have great power – it can destroy or revitalise. In today's society we can see water as a powerful force. Natural disasters always hit the headlines, floods and typhoons have a strong destroying power. This has surely been evident during 1998 with the power of El Nino in South America, and closer to home the Easter floods in the UK. We should never underestimate the destructive power of water. But what of water's revitalizing qualities?

The spiritualistic value of water has been documented throughout the centuries. Ancient Greek gods used water as an eternal life giver and, according to legend, the ancient priests of Egypt were delivered in water. Our own society and culture adopted a 'spiritualistic attachment' to water, with Christians being welcomed into the church through a baptism of water. Water has been documented as a feminine sign and it is this femininity that has been developed by those who use 'rebirthing' as described by Star (1986). This unique bond between water, birth and femininity has facilitated the phenomenon of rebirthing, the art and skill of regressing the mind and body in water. The concept of transcending to another spiritual level may be alien to many of us but 'floatation' tanks are now finding their way into today's fringe medicine. The strong influence of rebirthing was described by Rima Beth Star in *The Healing Power of Birth,* in which she writes about her own rebirthing and the influence it had on her second delivery, following the drowning of her first child. In the UK, not many couples or practitioners have followed this pathway, but occasionally I have encountered parents who have read about this work. My experience of rebirthing is purely theoretical: I have no attachment to this concept. Water is provided in my practice for relaxation with no conscious thoughts of its regressive power.

The 'Greek Goddess' scenario is perpetuated through some authors' work, including Odent (1990, 1994) who examines a symbolic relationship with water. Aphrodite, Goddess of Love, and Venus are both said to have been born from the foam of the waves. This attitude is said to prevail within certain parts of our society and it is apparent that some advertising agencies play on the impression of peace and tranquillity of water. Water can be portrayed as a wondrous scene of power or sensuality. Who has not watched the film *From Here to Eternity* and failed to be inspired by the crashing waves on the shore, but in the 1950s the director was obliged to cut the intimate scene. Latter day directors have more scope. *Fatal Attraction* and *Dirty Dancing*, both popular films, played on more explicit sexual overtones. Our attraction to water and sexuality or sensuality should, therefore, not be underestimated. This concept of 'attractive' water is even played out with the link some authors make between dolphins, the so-called water midwives and their telepathy with pregnant women.

Beyond the Blue (Cochrane *et al*, 1998) explores further the unique relationship between land and sea mammals. The dolphin as 'midwife' and 'teacher' is discussed, together with the mammal's unique ability to receive subtle energy forces from around them. This telepathy may be the reason why we, as land mammals, are attracted to the sea for its healing powers. Indeed it would appear that almsot every week we read stories of how children are taken to swim with dolphins in a controlled environment, in the hope of improving their own physical or mental ability.

Early documented work from Russia showed Tjarkovsky's fascination with dolphins.This was explored in Sidenbladh (1983). In 1992 this strong attachment to dolphins was followed by a team of mothers, accompanied by Dr Gowri Motha, an Obstetrician from Whipps Cross Hospital, London. The group of mothers were to have given birth in a private dolphin farm in Eilat, Israel. The project was not sanctioned by the Israeli government or medical personnel in the UK. Eventually only one waterbirth occurred secretly by a mother from East Sussex (Fox, 1992). The concept of this unique bond between dolphins and pregnant women, as identified by Tjarkovsky and Odent, is also being investigated in other parts of the world and with other disciplines.

During Tjarkovsky's first visit to the UK in 1989 his principle of water being 'the cradle of life on earth' was highlighted through his work in both water training and birth. His video of water training graphically portrayed the apparent trust that Russian women had in his ideas, allowing their babies to be submerged in ice-cold water. Here his work was highly criticised and the NSPCC went so far as to prevent his re-entry to the UK on the grounds of cruelty to children. His original beliefs of giving birth in water were based on his thoughts that, 'the sudden exposure at birth to the full force of gravity places a huge insult of oxygen on the sensitive brain functions.'

I have been unable to find any other professional who accepts or has evidence which substantiates his theories. These were cited in Ray (1985). Despite initial attempts to provide credence to his work, the lack of documented evidence will probably ensure that he remains on the fringe element of 'hydrotherapy'. Tjarkovsky's influence in modern-day practice should not, however, be undervalued. Like many pioneers in medicine, his skills and concepts are thought to be radical and controversial.

Leboyer's work, from which Tjarkovsky is said to have gained inspiration, could also have been classed in this category. In 1975 *Birth Without Violence* described the joys of gentle birth, topical in today's society, but in 1960 seen as radical. His description of using water as a healing therapy stimulates me to delve deeper into his work.

> *Water... this is where he has come from, and what he's known all his life. It's gentle, it's familiar. It is the very familiarity that in the end will completely calm him. It will be like meeting an old friend when one is far from home.*

Leboyer's work is well worth revisiting for its straightforward attitude towards gentle birth and using water immediately after birth. He stresses the need for a quiet, peaceful environment at the moment of birth. He believed that this slow stimulus to the baby's senses placed him or her in good stead for future development. Leboyer identifies birth as a momentous transition into a new world and that it is the gate through which he enters a new kingdom.

In today's society we have accepted the attitude that birth has a profound effect on mother and baby for their future bonding. Klaus and Kennell (1982) highlighted these issues and much of our present-day birthing practices are centred around these values and beliefs.

In 1970 Odent established his unit in Pithiviers, south of Paris, described in *Birth Reborn* (1984). Odent's emphasis on environment and care givers, revolutionised practice in western hospitals. He was one of the first to identify the importance of empowering women, to facilitate them to regain control over childbirth. In the film *Birth Reborn*, viewers were given the opportunity to see Odent at work, singing in parentcraft classes and setting the scene for natural birth. His first tentative steps towards using water for labour and eventually delivery were from the apparent attraction that women displayed towards water during labour. The early thoughts on water being a powerful therapy were at last being related by Odent to a physiological basis (reducing adrenergic secretions, promoting endorphin production and reducing sensory input). Odent (1984, p.46) continues:

Water can be as comforting as a lover, a mother or a midwife.

His philosophy to care is built on the premise that water provides a calm, reassuring environment that stimulates and enhances normal labour. Water labour and birth have now become the trademark of Odent, although this was not his original intention at Pithiviers. Water has been used at times when labour is long, or when the cervix is 6cm dilated, to enhance the uterine activity. Although now living and working in London, Odent has maintained his strong philosophy of empowering women and with his care women continue to have home waterbirths.

As Odent was developing his service, Michael Rosenthal in America was re-creating this relaxed and calm environment in his Family Birthing Centre, Upland California. Rosenthal's attitudes were similar to Odent. His centre offered women the opportunity to labour and deliver in a birthing centre with a holistic stance towards care. Two birthing tubs were available and widely used by the women in the centre. The family-centred approach was relatively unique in contemporary American society. High litigation and political pressures in the USA may have swayed women into believing big is beautiful (including large hospitals) and that childbirth can only be regarded as normal in retrospect.

Rosenthal could yet again be seen as being on the fringes of obstetric practice. The centre was attached to a hospital and this may have assisted him in developing a credible service. Hydrotherapy offered within the unit followed Rosenthal's belief that water offers a safe and calming environment in which to labour and deliver – indeed nearly 1,000 waterbirths had occurred prior to the unit closing in 1993. Women were willing to travel great distances to attend the centre, where they were assured of a calm and relaxed atmosphere, even in the entrance areas where a small fountain greeted them on arrival. The centre is more fully described in Chapter Four.

In the UK, as other pioneers were forging new skills and attitudes in obstetric practice, one shining light emerged. Roger Lichy, a GP in Penzance, Cornwall was developing a total concept of care. He already used homeopathy and complementary therapies in his practice. Lichy was already identifying a strong attraction to water and in *Katie's Birth* (shown on BBC television in 1988) the story was vividly unfolded in front of viewers. This was the first time that I had seen a waterbirth on television – in the tub that was carried around on the top of the GP's car! Once again, client demand had opened new horizons for consumers and care givers alike.

In *Waterbirth* (1990) Balaskas and Gordon write, 'Water may offer a seclusion from the hospital environment and a natural sanctuary in a homebirth.' This attitude to care during labour and delivery appears to mimic the skills and values of many practising midwives within the UK. Midwives are regaining their traditional craft, not always easy in today's ever changing health service and the historical background of medicalization (Clarke, 1993). The original, and some might say the lost concept of midwife meaning 'with woman' would seem to me to be encompassed in using hydrotherapy, returning the power to women and facilitating full involvement in care.

This newest ideal of empowerment is sweeping UK at the present time with 'Winterton' (1992) and *Changing Childbirth* (1993). Many maternity units today are attempting to introduce empowerment in its purest form – giving legal power to authorise. It is the women who have the power and now acknowledge their legal right to demand a change in service provision. A service which reflects a client-centred approach and is sensitive to change is nothing new. Odent (1984) summarised these ideas in writing:

> To sum up, privacy, intimacy, calm, freedom to labour in any position, and the helpful presence of midwives are crucial to a spontaneous first stage of labour.

How much more is this reflected than in waterbirth and its non-interventionist concept to caring. Two recent documents that have a profound effect on the way that waterbirths are viewed could be supported by the use of commissioning services in the new NHS.

In *Commissioning women centred maternity care* (RCN, 1996) the issue of responding to local need reflects how waterbirthing services could develop in light of consumer requests.

- *Consumer consultation.* What do women actually want for themselves and their babies?
- *Consultation with the maternity services liaison committee.* The multi-professional and consumer group can be useful supporters in developing a service.
- *Analysis of health, social, cultural and demographic data.* This is useful to understand whether there would be a demand for home/hospital service. Would women be willing to pay for liners or tub hire?
- *Identifying inequality of access to care.* Are all women able to access the service? Is written information available in other languages to reflect local populations?
- *Identifying gaps in the service.* Access to information and literature – are staff supported in offering waterbirths at home and hospital?
- *Targeting local priorities.* Resourcing a waterbirth service may need to be considered in the light of other requests for funding and time. Be creative in fundraising projects.
- *Developing strategies for future planning of services.* If water-birthing services are not possible at present, forward plan to the next financial year. Most business plans are designed six months in advance.

Women's views of maternity services are presented in *First Class Delivery* (1998). The use of water as a pain relief is discussed with other types of analgesia. It is interesting to note that only 6 per cent of women interviewed used water. This is compared to 76 per cent using entonox, 42 per cent using injectable analgesia and 27 per cent using epidurals. These figures could be used as a basis for each unit to analyse both present and future analgesia use. It would also be possible to assess any changes to analgesia use and the cost implications for maternity services.

The origins of hydrotherapy stem from promoting and restoring good health. Whilst there may be disagreements about water being self-indulgent, the basic assumption from Victorian times was that 'taking the waters' (internally or externally) was a good therapy. Water was seen as opposite ends of a continuum – stimulant versus relaxant, exercise versus rest (Inglis and West, 1983).

Hydrotherapy became particularly fashionable during the 18th century through Beau Nash and remained popular until the First World War. It lost its respectability and became known as a cure for insanity and of doubtful therapeutic value. By the time the NHS came into existence in 1948, the medical profession's attitude was that 'anything water could do, drugs could do better'. No free spa therapies were available within the UK after 1948, although they continued to flourish throughout Eastern Europe. They became the trademark for the affluent in communist countries. The magnificent natural wonder of the Turkish limestone cliffs at Pamukkale still attract thousands of visitors each year. The popularity of the pools is so great that the authorities are now thinking of making walkways to stop tourist erosion. In Germany spa towns have continued to flourish and still offer early morning warm-ups, exercises, massages, loofah baths and herbal wraps!

Evidence of the use of aromatherapy and, in particular, relaxing baths can be seen in any health or chemist shop today. Indeed, there appears to be few mental or physical ailments that do not have their own preparation on the shelves. *The Scented Bath*, (Riggs, 1991), is devoted to relaxation and relaxing baths. The book brings together:

twenty recipes for enchanting bathing rituals, each designed to create a certain mood, ease a specific problem or simply induce a sense of psychological and physical wellbeing.

Thalassatherapy has developed more slowly over the past 30 years and this sea therapy includes massage, baths of differing temperatures, underwater exercises, pressurised water jets and seaweed packs. Even in today's high tech society, the spa towns of Grofenburg in Austria and Spa in Belgium bear testimony to the use of these therapies.

Hydrotherapy's role in obstetrics is poorly documented, save for some references to Finnish women being taken to saunas for confinement (Nicol, 1975).

Conclusion

Finally, as you read other authors' work it is worth seeing why perhaps hydrotherapy is regaining popularity. Stanway (1979) writes:

> *Most often... I feel water therapy is beneficial because it is carried out by pleasant caring people, who together with the pampered atmosphere usually surrounding the therapy, induce a sense of mental wellbeing in the patient. Mental improvement in turn produces a reduction in anxiety and stress orientated symptoms and signs and he goes away feeling better... which is what all medicine is about.*

CHAPTER THREE

One unit's experience of waterbirth

Even for a unit that believes in freedom of choice, client participation and midwives working as autonomous practitioners, a waterbirth request was something new. It was late summer 1987 when Linda, a friend and professional colleague, approached me to see if I knew anything about waterbirth. One of her clients had seen a television report on the news about waterbirth in Russia and now finding herself pregnant wanted to know if this option was available in Maidstone. Even before the *Winterton Report* (1992) and *Changing Childbirth* (HMSO, 1993) we had always attempted to be sensitive to social change and proactive to new patterns of care. Attitudes to service provision and the way that women were involved in decision-making is reflected in Kitzinger (1987) and Huntingford (1985).

What followed was a frenzy of activity that consumed both midwives and the parents. A detailed account was written by Ford and Garland (1989) and Hughes (1989). This was to form the centre of the waterbirthing service at Maidstone and shows just how well consumers and professionals work together, given the right incentive. Although seen as a consumer-led development, it will become apparent as you read that it was the interest and 'trigger' from parents that forged the way. Several avenues needed to be tackled and each of us involved took a particular angle.

The first problem was that the maternity unit was designed in the late 1970s, when it was not really envisaged that women would be up and about in labour and there would be no need for bathrooms, just shower cubicles. The parents and midwives, therefore, set about attempting to find a suitable 'tub'. It was one month prior to the estimated date of delivery that finally the problem was resolved with a home-made tub. Designed and built by Mike Torode (the client's husband) the tub was portable and measured 6 x 3.6 x 1.8ft. It was made of white melamine and bolted together, with a groundsheet used as a liner. A car battery pumped the water out after use. There were a couple of dry runs using the tub, in which leaks were sorted out and it was brought to the maternity unit ready for the big day.

Looking back, the first tub is very similar to the portable baths now on the market, but in 1987 waterbirths were being undertaken in a wide variety of receptacles. Stories transpired about paddling pools, fish ponds and a 'skip', none of which seemed suitable to either our client or the maternity unit's structural engineers.

Having established that a tub was now available, Linda and I completed a literature search into waterbirth. We were greatly disappointed with the amount of material that was available. It soon became apparent that there was little written work and that as midwives if we were to fulfil our *Code of Practice* (UKCC, 1991) regarding 'acquiring competence in new skills' (p.6) other avenues would need to be sought.

It was therefore with great delight that we were put in contact with an independent midwife working on the south coast. Jill McKenna became our 'expert' and shared with us her experiences of water labour and birth. As a midwife, I was so impressed with the frankness and skill-sharing she offered us over the telephone that I decided to work with my maternity unit to set up our own workshops as soon as clinical experience became available. The information that Jill shared was fundamental in shaping the open access to clinical and theoretical input that started at Maidstone, within months of Chantelle's, and subsequently Bobby April's birth.

We attempted to contact other units offering waterbirth and very soon built up a good network with other departments and individual practitioners in a similar position to Maidstone. One article was highlighted as being of value to us. In 1983 Odent wrote about birth under water in Pithiviers, France. The article discussed some issues regarding the use of water in midwifery and obstetrics but did not give information about how to manage complications. Again these issues were discussed with Jill McKenna and are now shared with the reader in Chapter Ten.

The maternity unit's supervisor of midwives was involved from the beginning and, in the light of recent events in other units, this would appear vital. The Supervisor acted as a facilitator for information, steered us towards other resources and negotiated with other health professionals. As I have now become a supervisor, I realise just how important and fundamental this role was. It also became apparent that the Royal College of Midwives (RCM), and UKCC needed to be involved at the earliest opportunity. Supervision played a vital role in developing the service over the next year, as staff were introduced to the concept of water labour and birth.

Clinical scenario: supervision

Dawn

Linda and I decided that as this was our first waterbirth we would keep a daily diary. We hoped that this would encourage 'reflective practice' and act as a learning curve, for both the midwives directly involved and those who would skill share in the future. This diary also formed the basis for the article that was written and as an early means of evaluation (What would we do differently – second time around?).

When Dawn went into labour she contacted Linda, her community midwife. Her mother and husband both came in to be with Dawn. Whether it was her labour and delivery expectations, birth companions or known birth attendants that made Dawn's delivery so special is still not clear to us. But the birth of Chantelle remains in the memory of both Linda and myself even today.

Lyn

Within two months, the now famous or maybe one should say infamous, birthing tub was to be used again by another mother. Lyn had already booked a homebirth and on hearing about the hospital waterbirth enquired whether she could use the tub at home. Her daughter Bobby April was delivered safely and once again Lyn's birth experience was recorded in Hughes (1989).

Michelle

In this clinical case it was the first time that a previous caesarean section client had a waterbirth. The consultant, community midwife and supervisor spent time discussing and planning the birth. This multidisciplinary approach included Michelle who spoke about her wish to have a waterbirth with her second child but found this had not been possible within the unit's criteria. With her third pregnancy, she again spoke to her community midwife about this option. As supervisor, I was involved both in clinical and professional support. A joint decision was made that a rota between the community midwife and two supervisors would exist. In this way Michelle knew that one of these three would deliver her. A trusting and supportive environment was fostered, with Michelle gaining confidence from this system. For the midwives, it provided an opportunity to utilise the supervisors in their true professional role.

The waterbirth was a great success and there were no problems. I was on call the night Michelle went into labour. After a smooth and short labour, a gentle birth occurred with the delivery of a baby girl.

Following these birth experiences, it was decided that the maternity unit would like to offer this choice to all low risk women who came to Maidstone. It took a year from Chantelle and Bobby April's births to the opening of our 'Lagoon' room and a further year on for the 'Marine' room. During this time several more midwives showed an interest in joining what became a steering group for the project. Not all colleagues, however, were as keen as the steering group and we were surprised at some of the comments made during the early days. Looking back, it is apparent that most of these comments were based on professional concerns regarding accountability and acquisition of new skills.

Initially we set out to provide workshops for all staff within the maternity unit. This included all professionals, with special invites given to the medical staff. My colleagues and myself spent a great deal of time talking about the first two waterbirths and the benefits we considered this method offered Dawn and Lyn in labour and delivery. The local National Childbirth Trust (NCT) was approached early on, as it was clear that some fundraising would be required in setting the project up. It soon became a joint effort between professionals and consumers wishing to work together in offering this service to all mothers in Maidstone. The literature search that had already started was now extended and we involved our local medical library in the work. This has continued even today, with many articles being forwarded from both here and abroad. Links were established with Waterbirth International (now Global Maternal and Child Healthcare project). These links have played a vital

WATERBIRTH/LABOUR AUDIT FORM

Date:
_____

Mother's name and address

_____

Gravida:

Parity:
_____

Dilation on entering water.........cm
_____

Duration of labour:

1st stage timed from .../... hrs

2nd stage timed from .../... hrs

3rd stage timed from .../... hrs
_____

Duration of immersion:

Entered water at ....../...... hours

Left water at ....../...... hours
_____

Reason for leaving water
_____

Outcome of delivery
_____

Third stage management ❑ Dry ❑ Water
_____

Syntometrine given? ❑ Yes ❑ No
_____

Blood loss ❑ < 500mls ❑ > 500mls
_____

Perineum
_____

Apgar score .... 1min 5min
_____

Resuscitation required
_____

Baby to SCBU? ❑ Yes ❑ No
_____

Reason
_____

Method of feeding? ❑ Breast ❑ Formula
_____

Did mother attend aquanatal? ❑ Yes ❑ No
_____

Did mother attend waterbirth evening? ❑ Yes ❑ No
_____

Midwives' comments
_____

Parents' comments
_____

role in literature reviews, professional visits and skill sharing. Preparing for the development of this type of service was assisted by reading several text including *Birth Reborn* (Odent, 1984). This book shared the attitude to care of client choice and midwife autonomy, within an environment that facilitated active labour and delivery.

The maternity unit's supervisor became facilitator between the medical and managerial staff, who would need to be informed and involved in planning this facility. As already explained, the unit had a philosophy of proactive change and it was in this light that the option for water labour/birth was established. All health professionals who were likely to have contact with clients were involved, i.e. midwives, medics and health visitors. Others who soon became part of the 'team' were the building department and microbiology unit. Guidelines were drawn up as part of the planning for the use of the 'Lagoon' room (see Chapter Five).

Being aware of the need to audit and evaluate the service, senior staff designed two hand-held record forms, which all midwives were asked to complete along with the normal maternity records. These forms have been completed on all women who use the tubs for labour and/or delivery. An example is shown on page 33.

These forms have been evaluated and changes made in the light of clinical practice. For example, it became obvious that it was important to know the time that labour started, as well as the time that the woman actually entered the water. This gave a basis of the rate of cervical dilation following pain relief in water as a comparison with other forms of analgesia. I have also used the forms with a researcher as the basis for an article (Garland and Jones, 1994). We also noted that on most occasions the baby did not cry on immersion. This was recorded on the audit form – whether this is significant or not is thought to be an area of wider debate.

In the light of the *Midwives Rules* (UKCC, 1991, p.21) all records were kept as contemporaneously as possible and have not been destroyed, but stored by myself within a secure area.

Since the first waterbirths occurred, the maternity unit has implemented a computer records programme. As part of this system called 'Euroking', our computer midwife has written in a water labour/birth package. This has increased the audit provision and collection of objective data. As many units develop computer systems, the need to have clinical input is vital. It has been suggested that these systems are not always responsive to individual departmental needs but this was not our experience.

Following these waterbirths, it became apparent that a permanent waterbirthing facility would be required if the department was to offer this analgesia and delivery mode to all low-risk women. A description of the planning of the 'Lagoon' and 'Marine' rooms is recounted in Chapter Five.

Conclusion

This type of support and partnership in care became the goal post by which I set a standard for care at Maidstone. I was so impressed by the skill sharing offered by Jill McKenna that this shaped the waterbirth workshops now available. The vast number of visits and phone calls I have received have shown me that colleagues value this support. Continued meetings with both Dawn and Lyn and the children have shown me that not only have they grown up into normal healthy and mischievous little girls, but they have shared with their mothers a unique birth experience.

CHAPTER FOUR

International perspectives on waterbirth

The American connection

The American healthcare system often appears to UK practitioners to be unwieldy and cumbersome. It is interesting that in America healthcare is such big business. It is estimated to account for 14 per cent of the gross national income or $820 billion per year. Those who have private insurance schemes expect and get high standards of care, increased use of technology and short waiting times.

Healthcare in 1993 was given high status in President Clinton's first 100 days of office. Open access to insurance programmes and universal healthcare provision was seen as paramount. In a country in which administration accounts for 25 per cent of costs and healthcare is outside the scope of 14 per cent of Americans (some 36 million people) this parody of healthcare availability versus access seems ironical. This policy caused major problems for Clinton and has now been reviewed.

For many Americans the only access to healthcare is through the 'free clinic' system, of which only six existed in 1993. The federal system only provides emergency obstetric services and although used by many women, particularly the young, unemployed and those from minority groups, the 'free' system relies heavily on drug company donations for its resources. Within this type of society, inequalities in health are unfortunately bound to occur. This is reflected in the perinatal mortality rates in differing groups.

USA overall population	10:1,000
Caucasians	8.5:1,000
Ethnic minorities	17.6:1,000
UK figures as a comparison	8.9:1,000

(Crumble, 1993)

This inequality was described to me whilst visiting the USA. A typical scenario seen in emergency departments is of a woman arriving in labour with delivery imminent. She has had little or no antenatal care and once delivered will return home usually within hours. Postnatal care is almost non-existent and would for most women be too expensive.

Another factor to take into consideration in the USA is the current legal situation. Practising 'defensive' obstetrics means that in some maternity units the LSCS rate is running at 25 per cent and that in some hospitals childbirth is only seen as normal in retrospect. Practitioners are also experiencing increasing difficulties in getting insurance cover. This is particularly apparent in California where some midwives are now practising with no insurance cover. Overlaying these issues is the social melting pot that is unique to the States. Over many years the healthcare needs of minority and transient populations have largely been ignored. All of these factors are being taken into account as the American College of Nurse Midwifery strives to develop more doctorate and Master programmes. Midwives view childbirth as normal and are attempting to reverse the current trends in high tech, expensive, hospital-based care.

The training programmes may well differ from the UK but the fundamental theory and practice interface exists, although these Nurse Midwives have a wider remit into gynaecology and women's health. Regaining a foothold in pregnancy and childbirth is paramount for the midwives, who often have to gain 'privileges' to work in hospitals (i.e. have access to hospitals for delivery beds). It was during the late 1980s and in this climate of change that I was first introduced to midwives in Ohio; these links having developed into a unique bond which still exist today. The University of Case Western Ohio had some time ago identified the value of Nurse Midwives and in their report (1992) wrote:

They provide personalised and comprehensive care with emphasis on teaching... nurse midwives encourage expectant parents to participate actively in all aspects of their care and to prepare themselves physically and emotionally for the birth experience.

This attitude to care is gradually gaining momentum as women and professionals identify the value of midwifery with its unique bond between parents and midwives. It will not be an easy struggle. American legislation may need to be altered to allow all 52 states to have the opportunity to train and permit midwives to practice.

During this time the rebirthing phenomena evolved and waterbirths started to be practised. To a rebirther the thought of underwater birth appears to be a 'natural' progression. Ray (1985) describes the actual process of rebirthing and the positive move to waterbirths, thus encompassing Leboyer's work. To those who believe in the strong spiritual and psychological overlay at the time of birth, this gentle attitude towards labour and delivery is very important. The first two waterbirths in the US are described by Ray, writing about Jia and Patrick Lighthouse (who delivered without medical support) and Rima Beth Star who delivered in Austin Texas.

Other practitioners started to get interested and Karil Daniels became involved in home waterbirths, utilizing visualization and meditation. Working in partnership with other 'enlightened' practitioners waterbirth slowly started to develop in the USA (Daniels, 1988; 1989). Out of this pioneering work Waterbirth International (WBI) was formed. It was originally based in Santa Barbara, California, and now in Portland, Oregon. A more relaxed medico-legal, political and social structure encouraged WBI to move in 1992. In a supporting statement from WBI they write:

> WBI support... attitudes and practices which acknowledge the fact that birth is not a medical event and which fulfils the needs of a woman as they perceive them.

WBI assist in disseminating information and questionnaires regarding the use of water tubs. They hire out a portable 5ft diameter tub and have a comprehensive database. WBI's founder Barbara Harper has personal experience of waterbirths, which she openly shares with consumers and professionals (Harper, 1990).

In 1992 I was able to visit Santa Barbara and had the opportunity to access their database and forge links with worldwide waterbirth colleagues. One of these contacts was with Michael Rosenthal and his unique Family Birthing Centre, Upland California (FBC). The unit opened in January 1985 and during the next eight years experienced nearly 1,000 waterbirths. Rosenthal had worked in traditional units but was keen to establish a unit that followed a 'birth without rules' philosophy. Rosenthal's attitudes are simple. He believed in 'mothering' women in labour, whether that was by a family member or birth attendant. Through this attitude he aimed to reduce professional control and increase the empowerment of women. The medico-legal society within which Rosenthal practised had, he believed, made it difficult to change and that practice had moved too far down the medical model. The FBC offered a balance between low-risk care, in a relaxed atmosphere, with a traditional

Table 4.1: Family birthing centre – upland California

Client group	*85 per cent Caucasian* *12 per cent Hispanic*
Cost of service	*$1600–$1900*
Care givers	*Obstetrician/Midwives* *Labour Nurses*
Tubs available	*Two fibreglass* *150 gallons*
Protocol for use	*Normality/low-risk* *Available for VBACs* *Cervical dystocia*
Primip:multip ratio	*50:50*
Additives to water	*None*
Water temperature	*Maternal comfort (32-37°C)*
Monitoring	*Hand held doppler*
Third-stage management	*Dry land – physiological*
Outcomes	*2/3 women deliver in water* *1700 labours* *900 waterbirths* *Apgars = SVDs* *> tears 1st and 2nd degree* *No 3rd or 4th degree* *One minor infection* *High percentage breastfeed*
Cleaning/audit	*Cleaned with Benzalkonium chloride* *Swabs taken*

hospital only a stone's throw away. He believed that the Nurse Midwives played a vital role in the statistical outcomes in the unit. They certainly appeared very impressive.

SVD   86.5 per cent
LSCS   8-9 per cent (USA 26-30 per cent)

Whilst it was true that Rosenthal's clients were fee-paying, the cost ($1600–$1900) was still said to be a third cheaper than traditional maternity care. The fee included prenatal, labour and – fairly unique in the USA – postnatal follow-up. The client group were from a wide cross-section of American society and were willing to travel many miles to deliver at the centre.

American society has, Rosenthal believes, the unique ability to 'hybridise', i.e. take things apart and put it back together. He designed a unit where all the elements for low-risk care were available, including two birthing tubs. During my visit in 1992 I completed a short survey of practice, the details are shown in Table 4.1.

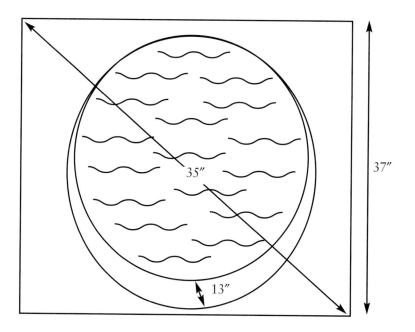

Fig. 4.1: Upright tub – top view

Table 4.2: Natural birthing centre, Culver City, Los Angeles

Client group	*Mixed class and cultures*
Cost of service	*$3900*
Care givers	*Midwives*
Tubs available	*One oval 110 gallons* *One upright 50 gallons* *Both fibreglass*
Protocol for use	*Normality*
Primip:multip ratio	*50:50*
Additives to water	*None*
Water temperature	*100°C measured with thermometer*
Monitoring	*Hand held doppler*
Third-stage management	*Physiological on dry land*
Outcomes (1991)	*50 per cent women deliver in water* *148 waterbirths* *Apgars = SVD* *> lacerations* *Infections – none*

Finally Rosenthal (1991) writes:

> *Warm water immersion can best be understood in this context...*
> *which views birth as a normal biological process, not as an illness*
> *or procedure... thus the practitioner who embraces this approach*
> *should be prepared to play a secondary role in childbirth,*
> *informing women of their options and supporting their decisions.*

This attitude to care is also reflected at the Natural Birthing Centre
(NBC) Culver City, Los Angeles. Here Nancy McNeese and her
colleagues have established a low-risk centre run by midwives. The
centre 'books' clients who have no adverse medical history and no
known obstetric complications. They have a strict protocol for referral
and transfer to the nearest hospital. Parents attend for antenatal,
intrapartum and a short postnatal stay (usually 2–3 hours). Clients are
encouraged to attend parentcraft classes and to stop smoking or drinking
as a prerequisite for attending the centre. Two birthing tubs are available
for the women to use during labour and delivery. One is a traditional

shape and depth, whilst the other could only be described as an 'upright' tub. Tabulated details of the Centre are shown in Table 4.2.

The NBC states that they believe water is merely an alternative type of care, that the issues it raises are more about a woman's right to choose a physically and psychologically safe and comfortable way to give birth. Here the birth process is seen as a shared responsibility and that clients have the right to choose where to have their babies born as well as how. Nancy McNeese summarises by writing,

> *This right implies responsibility, and the place where a woman gives birth can be totally safe only when she bears her share of the responsibility for the normal natural process.* (McNeese, 1988)

Another pioneering and well supported unit is Monadnock Community Hospital, Peterborough, New Hampshire. The results of their work, offered as a 'gentle' choice for women, and not as they describe a 'lofty' goal is discussed by O'Connell 1998. I have visited this unit several times

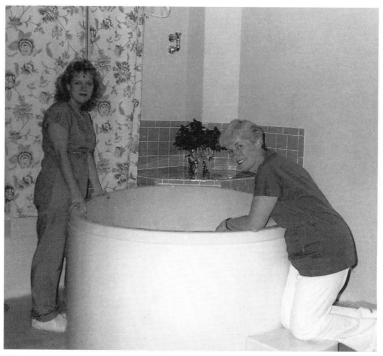

Fig 4.2: Birthing pool and staff at Monadnock Community Hospital, Peterborough, New Hampshire USA

and find their attitude to care and support of women's right to choose is refreshing in the USA where the medical mode of birth has so often been portrayed as the norm.

The European connection

The most important unit that came to the notice of Europeans was that in Pithiviers. Odent's unit, situated about 50 miles south of Paris, is a public hospital serving a mixed urban and rural population. Prenatal care was provided at the hospital and parenthood classes were conducted with the emphasis on partnership. There were opportunities to see around the unit and gather around the piano with all the family. Delivery occurred in whatever position or place the mother found comfortable and within this environment Odent found many women attracted to water. Obstetrics at Pithiviers evolved from these early beginnings (Odent, 1981).

In the coastal town of Ostende, Belgium, waterbirths have been undertaken for the past ten years in the Henri Serruys hospital. The unit is situated in the centre of Ostende and is a traditional unit, except for one fundamental issue. Herman Ponette, obstetrician and waterbirth pioneer has developed a service that is fairly unique in Belgium. The clients that come to Ostende are seeking the chance to use the waterbirthing tubs and his attitude to care. Women are prepared to travel 100 km from Brussels to deliver at Ostende, although Belgium is fairly lucky as there are four other units that also undertake waterbirths. Despite initial criticism from other professionals, Ponette continued with his work. The midwives and obstetricians work very closely together, skill-sharing clinical experience, although no formal training takes place. Ponette has a non-interventionist attitude to care and his figures are certainly impressive.

LSCS rate

Ponette	5-6%
Henri Serruys hospital	7%
Belgium	12-14%

Herman Ponette is unusual, in that he aims to add salt (freeze-dried sea water) to the tubs to an isotonic concentration, similar to amniotic fluid. Antenatal preparations are run through Aquarius, a symbiotic relationship existing where one appears to feed off the other. This antenatal preparation may be one reason why Ponette has a 60 per cent waterbirth rate.

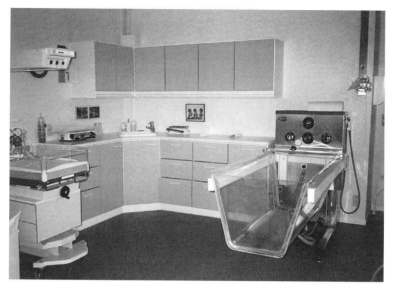

Fig. 4.3: Birthing tub – Henri Serruys Hospital, Ostende, Belgium

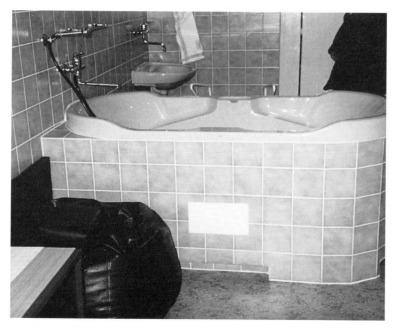

Fig. 4.4: Waterbirthing suite – Vrchalabi, Czech Republic

Aquarius has an antenatal preparation programme that includes swimming and relaxation, which promotes mental and physical wellbeing. The details of my visit to Henri Serruys Hospital, Ostende, Belgium in November 1994 are shown in Table 4.3.

Studies undertaken in Europe

In 1987 Gillot de Vries *et al* studied the experience for women who used warm water tubs during labour in a unit in Brussels. Most of the women believed that the bath was a positive idea.

- The water seemed to bring a better level of consciousness during delivery.
- The women felt more relaxed and less anxious.
- The women were more receptive to their babies.
- The researchers expected an improved establishment in mother-child interaction.

A study in Denmark was reported by Lenstrup *et al* (1987). In this study 88 women bathed in a warm tub for periods from half an hour up to two hours in the first stage. A control group of 72 women fulfilling the same criteria were used to assist measurements of mean pain scores and cervical dilation.

- Mean pain scores were higher in the bath group.
- The non-bath group had an increase use of stimulation.
- No differences were observed in operative delivery, perineal trauma, bleeding or neonatal outcomes.

Other studies worth reading include Doniec-Ulman *et al* (1987) and Gradert *et al* (1987). A final European perspective is that voiced by Zimmermann, Huch and Huch (1993). They write:

> *Waterbirths have gradually become more popular in industrialised countries during the last decade... However there is a great lack of scientific data. Several neonatal deaths are reported during uncontrolled waterbirths. Based on the knowledge available to date, physiological and general considerations, waterbirths must be classed as a type of obstetrical management.* **Waterbirths should thus be restricted to centres with adequate medical assistance and only in controlled studies.** (My emphasis)

Table 4.3: Henri Serruys Hospital, Ostende, Belgium

Client group	*Mixed social classes*
Cost of service	*20,000 BF*
Care givers	*3 Obstetricians* *Midwives*
Tubs available	*2 perspex*
Protocol for use	*All comers* *Tubs available for Twins/Breech* *Previous LSCS*
Primip:multip ratio	*30:70*
Additives to water	*Salt added to amniotic fluid* *isotonic volume*
Water temperature	*36-37°C measured and recorded* *Thermostat control on tub*
Monitoring	*Hand held doppler following base CTG*
Third-stage management	*Physiological – dry land*
Outcomes	*Length of labour reduced in* *Multips by 50%* *Primips 30%* *Perineal trauma* *No increase in tears* *Small episiotomies performed* *Apgar scores similar to other* *Post-partum haemorrhage increased if* *placenta delivered in water*

I believe this attitude shows just why so many medical practitioners are against waterbirths – they are just not in control! Hopefully since the first International Waterbirth Conference at Wembley in April 1995, these attitudes will gradually alter. (See Appendix VII for countries practising waterbirths.)

Since the first international conference, more European work has become available in the UK. In an interview with Dr Rockenschaub from Vienna, Beverley Beech reported on how Dr Rockenschaub's unit first undertook waterbirths in 1986 and that since this date more than 2,000 waterbirths have occurred. One of the most impressive issues raised is the very low

Table 4.4: Birth Unit, Vienna, Austria

	Dry land birth	First stage use of water	*Number of women (in per cent)* Waterbirth
Total	37	52	11
Use of analgesia:			
None	66	33	67
Pethidine	0	3	0
Homeopathy	21	37	25
LSCS rate:	0.87	2.83	0
Perineum:			
Intact	31	29	52
Sutured	69	71	48

LSCS rate (1.05 per cent), which is considered to be the result of a combined attitude to care, intervention and support during labour. (Beech 1996).

During a visit to the Czech Republic in 1997, I was fortunate enough to lecture with Dr Volker Korbei, from this Viennese unit. He further explained the unit's statistics, which do need to be borne in mind when reviewing the LSCS rate. Firstly, the unit is mainly private, with middle to upper class women. They have three delivery rooms and have approximately eight births per day. However, the figures discussed at this conference were even more impressive (see Table 4.4). Like many statistics it is important not to take these in isolation; it is important to be aware of the risk category of women at the unit. However, as time continues, this type of work may become more accessible to UK practising midwives and thus the opportunity to evaluate the statistics. This conference was published in 1998 by Hlavackova. Future work by the hosts of this conference (Dr Libor Kavan and Czech midwives) is eagerly awaited, since it will add more support to the growing body of evidence building up around the world on waterbirths.

Evidence from Sweden by Eriksson *et al* (1997) suggests that it is preferable that women do not enter the water until they have reached 5cm. Many units are now moving away from a set starting cervical dilation for entering the water. However, there is still a need to ensure that women are in strong established labour, and that both the nature and time of contractions is carefully observed by the midwife, to ensure that labour does not slow or alter when in the water for the first hour. In the author's experience, if this is undertaken, it is clinically easier to assess if women have or have not entered the water too early. Other European centres can be read about in *Waterbirth Unplugged*, 1996, by Beverley Beech.

Conclusion

The American and European systems of care may well be different to that which is offered in Britain but as a midwife the fundamental attitude that prevails is the same. We are seen as supporters of women in the provision of options and empower them to make informed choice in all aspects of care. Whatever system one works within, the philosophy of holistic and proactive care means that families can achieve a sensitive and pleasurable birth experience.

CHAPTER FIVE

Setting up a waterbirthing facility

Whilst other units, both in the UK and abroad, were starting up waterbirth centres, my own unit decided to take its first tentative steps towards a permanent waterbirthing facility. The maternity unit is within a NHS hospital situated outside the county town of Maidstone. Like many units 'conceived' in the late 1970s and early 1980s, the concept of labouring women being up and mobile was not really in the minds of the designers. Consequently, the unit was built in the style of an active managed labour ward with shower rooms but no baths. Many new units have been built since 1990 and these have included water tubs as an integral part of the design. Liverpool maternity unit and Caroline Flint's birthing centre are but two, with very different scopes for care. This change in unit design and attitudes towards the use of water, reflect care as encompassed by the *Winterton report* (House of Commons Health Committee, 1992) where it was written:

> *We recommend that all hospitals make their policy to make full provision, whenever possible, for women to choose the position that they prefer for labour and birth, with the option of a birthing pool where this is practicable.*

Like many units who started waterbirths in the 1980s, our first tub was homemade, since those now on the market were not yet available. The 'Heath Robinson' approach seemed to work well for our first two deliveries but the tub, along with other basic equipment, was not going to be suitable long-term. Some equipment was not even available on the

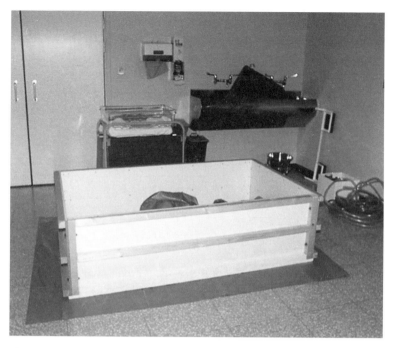

Fig. 5.1: Homemade tub designed by Mike Torode

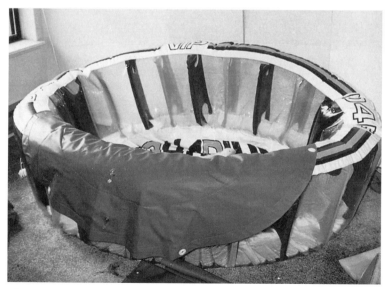

Fig. 5.2: Home birthing pool – USA style!

market at all – underwater monitoring was undertaken with a hand held doppler covered by a glove or condom! This was neither personally or professionally acceptable and was one issue reviewed very early on.

The first tub was designed by Mike Torode and Figure 5.1 shows the original tub set up at Maidstone Hospital. Its main problem was that being made of wood, the tub was rather heavy and there were concerns expressed about the weight on the labour ward floor. Our criteria for a permanent tub was that it would be easily available, cost-effective to install and easy to maintain. Since the first two waterbirths occurred, many companies have set about designing portable and permanent tubs. A list of companies is available in the Useful Addresses section in Appendix VI.

In 1989 the maternity unit redesigned its first birthing tub with the manufacturers Glass Fibre Mouldings. The 'aurora' lagoon bath measures 2,200cm long, 1,050cm wide and 460-680cm deep. It holds 187 gallons of water and weighs 1,870lbs when full. The design reflects several factors that were of concern to mothers and midwives with the first tub. A non-slip base was moulded in, and the tub contains a seat area and a 'well' part for squatting deliveries. The unit also built a plinth around the tub at three different heights on which the midwives kneel for labour and delivery (cushions are also provided). One feature which has proved invaluable is the more acute angled back. Usually baths are at 45° to the horizontal. The aurora is at 55° and appears to have overcome several comments by mothers regarding back support. This change in angle is to take into consideration the altered spinal posture in pregnancy.

It is worth investigating all of the tub options in portable and permanent tubs prior to purchasing. Size and cost may also play a part in choice. You should also consider safety aspects, hygiene or liner use and support for the woman in the water.

The aesthetic qualities of the waterbirthing room should be considered; some units have developed rooms which reflect the 'watery' theme. At Maidstone we have two rooms – the lagoon and marine rooms, which both have underwater murals painted on their walls. This relaxing theme was described by Blair Myers (1989) and highlights general thoughts on the aesthetic qualities, which are thought to be so important. The rooms also have soft furnishings, which complement the surroundings, together with dimmed lights to soothe the environment even more. At home you may wish to use protected candles to obtain the desired effect (I saw this used very effectively in a birthing centre in America). It is important to have access to large towels and gowns, which can be warmed under the radiant heater or radiators at home. Sometimes mothers can become chilled after the birth and, of course, it is important to keep the baby warm after delivery.

Other considerations include the heating, lighting and ventilation of the room. It is important to have a warm, well-ventilated area that is comfortable for parents and midwives. Beanbags and cushions certainly make life more comfortable for everyone and the availability of several chairs or stools of differing heights assist midwives in adopting positions for labour or delivery. Whether at home or in hospital you will also wish to ensure that you have easy access to a call bell system. At home this may mean telephone availability, and in hospital, a buzzer.

Planning a home waterbirth may necessitate hiring a portable birthing tub. There are many such companies now on the market, with a wide range of tubs available. Parents and professionals should take several issues into account when choosing which tub to hire. These include:

- Size and weight of tub. Where in the room will it be placed?

- Cost of hire. Is this for a four-week period, with extra charges for every day overdue? Or, is the tub a set price until you deliver? Are there charges involved in delivering the pool to your home?

- What is included in the hire charge? Do parents have to purchase any extras (see homebirth checklist)?

- Have local midwives had any experiences with tubs? If so, which do they believe are appropriate?

Hiring a birthing pool is an expensive issue and so great thought should be given to making the decision about which tub to hire. Discussion with local mothers and midwives who have had previous experience may assist with the choice. Some entrepreneurial maternity units now hire out their own birthing pools as another option for local mothers. Setting up as a business has several advantages. Firstly, access at a local level for mothers may reduce the cost of hiring. Midwives may feel more comfortable with a pool that they already know and are used to setting up, which may assist practice.

Midwives may be required to establish local demand for the pool; this could be achieved by advertising locally or by carrying out surveys at parentcraft sessions. It may, of course, be that mothers are coming through to midwives actually asking for pool hire. Whatever avenue is found to establish and purchase a pool, it is vital that a review is caried out of advertising, the appropriate local cost for hire and contracting of the service.

Whether the mother hires the pool from an individual or a company, several issues may need to be considered. These broadly fall into three main areas: practical/clinical; professional support; and setting up the pool at home. These issues should all be covered by a midwife during pregnancy (I usually undertake this at approximately 36 weeks). Following a home visit, a back-up letter is sent to the parents confirming what had been discussed at the earlier meeting. This system appears to work very well when both parents are seen. As a result of using it I have not encountered any problems during twelve years of home waterbirths (see Appendix IV).

Practical issues

Reasons for transfer to hospital
This may be based on local policy and/or professional recommendations. These areas should always be discussed with both parents and be clearly documented.

Equipment carried by community midwives
Homebirth bag - specialised equipment carried by the community midwife (doppler, sieve, water thermometer).

When to enter and leave tub
Many midwives do not have a set dilation at which point the mother may enter the water. Instead, each mother and labour is reviewed individually. However, mothers should be aware of some evidence (see Chapter Nine) which suggests early water use may slow or stop the labour. In clinical practice I have found that most primigravida women enter the water at 3/4cm, whilst multigravid women enter at 4/5cm. However, I have used water at 1cm and 10cm. When women enter the water early it is paramount that the nature of the contractions is evaluated for the first hour after immersion. This clinical evaluation is based on palpation of contractions, timing and strength, mothers' perception of contraction and pattern (i.e. change over one hour).

Leaving the water

In my experience this is based on three main reasons:

- Maternal request, i.e. further analgesia.
- Fetal compromise, i.e. meconium or changes to fetal heart rate.
- Failure to progress in labour.

There do, however, appear to be a small number of women who seek 'terra firma' to deliver on, and of course, where water labour/birth is supported this does not cause any conflict.

Guidelines for practice/physiological third stage

Many issues need to be considered when health assessing the woman's choice for physiological versus active third stage. This includes in water or out, since the early theoretical risk of water embolism has been dispelled (both by clinical practice and discussion with physiologists).

- The woman's antenatal history should be reviewed, with any risk factors noted. The last Hb check should be assessed and also whether she has had prolonged low haemoglobin levels.
- Previous third stage problems and management should be reviewed if the mother has delivered before.
- Review the nature of the labour, length of both latent and active, and whether she has had any other analgesia, i.e. pethidine prior to entering the water.
- The nature of the contractions in second stage should be assessed. Has the active part of second stage been long?

Find out the woman's choice for delivery of the placenta, ensuring that both she and her partner fully understand and consent to this choice. I always document this in the notes, particularly as the ways the third stage is conducted, i.e. active versus physiological are so different. I ensure women understand that with physiological, the third stage may take longer. In my experience the average length of time is 40 minutes, but I have known of 5 minute to 2 hour third stages.

If the woman chooses active management, she will need to leave the water, or have the tub drained immediately after the baby's birth, to allow an oxytocic to be given and for the cord to be clamped and cut without delay. This, of course, radically alters the first few minutes of interaction between mother and baby – an interaction which mothers often wish to have with a waterbirth.

Finally, the midwives' own skills with third stage management need to be considered. We may need to 'relearn' the art of physiological third stage, and avail ourselves to education. A very useful reference is that by Rogers *et al* 1998.

Care of other children

I always remind parents about the need to ensure that any other children who are in the household have a birth companion to look after them. The health and safety issues of having a large pool of water in the house, are also discussed. These same sort of principles could equally apply to any animals (who are also attracted to water).

Professional support

Calling of community team

It is of course vital that the parents know how to summon help and when to call the community team. Whilst this will differ between units, the principles of contact numbers and access to appropriate levels of support are paramount. If one community midwife is specifically 'on call' for this mother, has an out of hours service been discussed? What if the midwife is not available? And is vicarious liability cover (when not on duty) covered?

Profiles of teams

If the midwives work in a team (whatever sort of team that is in today's NHS) then a team profile is useful to parents. This may include a brief introduction to each midwife, with emphasis given to those midwives who have expertise in home waterbirths. This introduction is important since parents will often ask about experienced midwives and how 'cover' for home waterbirths is arranged. A network of support and expertise should be agreed at local level.

Ambulance response times

In each area, midwives should be aware of how long an ambulance response time is for each locality. Response times will vary, and if mother/baby are not in any danger other options could be explored. Is it feasible to bring the woman into hospital by her partner's car? When would you advise admission? Not only should these issues be discussed, but they should be recorded. (See Appendix IV.)

Waterbirth parents evening

If a waterbirth evening or educational session is available locally, I always ensure that parents are aware of this. There are of course many commercial companies who run parents evenings (for example, Active Birth Centre and Splashdown).

Role of Supervisor of Midwives

This will obviously be different for each area. However, as the East Herts scenario appeared to show, good clear verbal and written communication is essential between all those involved in a waterbirth at home. The supervisor may give practical/clinical support or expertise and act as a resource professionally. Whatever role the supervisor has, it is paramount that this is communicated to the midwives actually attending the home waterbirth (Does the supervisor wish to be informed antenatally, or called when the woman goes into labour?)

Setting up the pool at home

Water tub hire – private company

There are many private companies who now hire out birthing tubs; details are usually held locally. The local hospital may also hire out their own tub. Both of these options can be investigated. It is very helpful if the team of midwives who are going to provide care actually know which tub the parents are hiring, as there are many styles and types now on the market. Familiarity supports practice!

Health and safety issues

The main health and safety issues are governed by COSHH regulations 1999. Water and electricity do not mix, and it is just as important to observe this principle in the home as in hospital. If parents are using a small room to place the tub in, it is suggested that they purchase 'baby proof' plastic covers for all electrical sockets. These act to stop water humidity entering any sockets and as a reminder prior to plugging in any electrical equipment. It is also important to remember that expensive stereo and TV sets would be greatly damaged if water gets near to them. I usually suggest to partners that this type of equipment is moved away from the tub.

Structural/insurance details

During the home interview, I always suggest parents check their home insurance. Whilst I have never heard of any pool leaking (nor exploding as in the television series *Men Behaving Badly*) the tiny risk should be stated. Structurally, most modern day properties seem able to deal with the weight of a pool. It has been my experience only to be cautious with very old cottages! In these situations the downstairs rooms usually have solid floors and thus do not present any problems. Birthing pools have certainly been used in old and new, one-storey and high-rise flats without any recorded problems.

Partner's role and responsibility

When planning a home waterbirth, it is vital that the birth companion and partner (or whoever is going to set up the pool) is present when discussing their role and responsibilities. I ensure that I visit parents, usually in the evenings (or weekend, if required), to discuss the pool positioning in the home. Areas to be discussed include: ensuring the tub is accessible both for filling and emptying; ensuring adequate water supply; and that all equipment is set up prior to encouraging the woman to enter the pool. I stress that it is the partner's responsibility to care for the pool and that the midwives are there to care for the woman and not the pool!

Setting and collecting tub/dry run

Pools may be delivered or collected depending on where the parents are hiring from. I always suggest that the pool should be in the home from 38 weeks (usually a hire period is for 4 weeks). A dry run appears logical in order to work out how long the pool takes to set up, its positioning in the room and how long it takes to fill.

Basic equipment for water labour/births

- Water thermometer – we use an aquarium thermometer, as these are cheap, plastic and sterilizable. They also have a small suction cap which can stick to the base or side of the tub.
- Plastic sieve or fish net – same principles as above. This is needed to sift out any debris (which in my experience is minimal).
- Large towels and gowns.
- Step for access to tub or plinth if plumbed in.
- Hand held fans – the room may still become very warm despite ventilation.
- Cleaning materials or liners for portable tubs.
- Long gloves or sleeves for birth attendant.

Monitoring equipment is now more widely available than when I started water labours/births in 1989. Companies have taken on board the areas of concern that midwives have expressed, namely that an audible fetal heart sound and possibly digital display are vital. Company details are listed in the Useful Addresses section in Appendix VI. The days of monitoring with a hand held doppler covered by a glove or condom will, I believe, soon be obsolete. The benefits of being able to monitor totally submerged means that there is less disturbance to the mother.

Fundraising for your own 'lagoon' room may take some innovative thoughts and planning. We are all aware that funding is often a problem and this service may be seen to absorb vital resources. I would, therefore, suggest that you plan a high profile fundraising project. Get local consumer groups involved and seek media coverage. The midwives and parents in Maidstone undertook a joint project and did a sponsored army assault course at the local army barracks. It was not only a great way of raising money but did a great deal for team spirit, built on community links and was good fun.

I estimated that the lagoon room cost approximately £1,500 due to changes to lighting, plumbing, ventilation and tub purchase. Once installed and set up, the ongoing costs are very small and consist really of replacing thermometers, and so on. Minimal costs will occur as tap washers need replacement, but I have found that most expenditure is small compared with other service provision. One comment that has been voiced is that water labour/birth is elitist and only available to a select few. Whilst this is partly true, access is dependent upon local midwives and hospitals and tubs are far more widely available than they were a few years ago. The cost issue is often posed as a concern. One way to measure water's effectiveness is to cost per unit of analgesia (Table 5.1). These costings are purely based on the dose cost of analgesia and not on start up or personnel costs, i.e. purchasing TENS or tubs and anaesthetists' time.

Table 5.1: Costing per unit of analgesia (£)

Pethidine	0.14
Meptid	0.82
TENS battery	1.00
Epidural marcaine 5%	1.27
Aurora birthing tub	0.85

When setting up a waterbirth facility a variety of professionals may need to be included from the outset. One of these is the microbiology department. At Maidstone, our infection control nurse was involved from the beginning and was instrumental in drawing up a cleaning policy. The unit has strict cleaning guidelines. For example, the bath is cleaned daily as part of the domestic services and after each use. The most fundamental part of this cleaning is to allow the tub to dry in between uses. At home, it is important that the parents follow the manufacturers cleaning instructions and use a new disposable liner with each client. Some problems have been highlighted in the press regarding infection. Most of these reports have been with regard to cleansing of portable tub hoses (Hilson, 1994; Rawal, 1994). It is important that only essential equipment is kept in the room and that is does not become a dumping ground for other equipment.

Known active hepatitis B or HIV carrier mothers may be actively discouraged from entering the water. It is generally thought that in the amount of water and temperature variants that both of these viruses, which are vulnerable, would be disseminated. It is further thought that these would not, therefore, place mother, baby or midwife at any greater risk than on dry land. Policies should already exist within your department or practice for blood spillages and equipment cleaning in these situations. Health and safety issues are often addressed through local policies and help may be assisted by Royal College of Midwives stewards.

There have been several developments since this book was first published regarding HIV and hepatitis carriers. Firstly, during 1995/6 a London hospital announced that they would be asking all mothers wishing to use the pool to have HIV testing. (Knowsley 1995, Day and Ridgeway *et al* 1996). This caused the national and professional press to respond, and an expert group met under the auspices of the Terence Higgins Trust. Several issues arose and these are drawn together below for the reader to review. Interestingly, some three years later this hospital published their results (Forde *et al*, 1999).

Assessing the risk of HIV and hepatitis

- Risk needs to be assessed and balanced in light of current statistics. See Department of Health document April 1998.

- Risk needs to be assessed with regard to current screening policies and available counselling, support and referral.

- Current 'window' for testing of three months makes testing all women difficult. Testing may take several hours, but in most centres it takes several days to receive results. So impractical to test when in early labour.

- All clients should be treated with universal precautions, i.e. long sleeves or gauntlet gloves should be available.

- Cleaning requirements for tubs and equipment should be undertaken in light of local policy or company instructions.

- All equipment should be sterilised/cleaned/disposable.

- Both viruses are fragile, but can survive outside the body in the right environment. However, waterbirths are a non touch technique. An underwater monitor can be given to mother, thereby reducing the risk to midwife. The water volume may dilute red blood cells. Blood clots should be sieved out to avoid contamination.

- Infectivity is dependent on the quality and quantity of the virus (direct inoculation or mucosa contact with birth attendant).

- Routine swabs from pools may assist in defining a cleaning policy.

- No delivery can be totally 'risk free'. However, risk assessment and management can reduce risks to midwives, mothers and newborns. Forde *et al* (1999, p 171) conclude: *no increased risk of bacterial infection to mother or baby was demonstrated by this study*. There was no serious neonatal morbidity, but close monitoring is important. A protocol for maternal, fetal and neonatal observation is suggested. A randomised study comparing waterbirth with 'dry' land birth is long overdue.

Many of these issues are being or indeed have been addressed by experienced waterbirthers for many years.

Issues to review

- *Backache or injury.* I have not heard of any back injuries at Maidstone in seven years. A minimal handling policy means that you should not be leaning over the tub for any length of time (see Appendix V).

- *Water spillage.* This can occur as the woman steps out of the tub. All water should be cleared up as soon as possible.

- *Use of electrical equipment.* In Great Britain it is not possible to have water and electricity mixing in one room (see regulations for electrical installation (Institute of Electrical Engineers, 1991)). In units or homes where this is not practical or possible, one solution is to cover all electrical points with childproof covers. Brightly coloured covers mean that it is very obvious if the covers are not in place and also act as a reminder prior to removing them and plugging in electrical equipment. Fetal heart monitors and cassette players should be battery operated to overcome any potential hazard.

- *Scalding with hot water.* COHSE regulations state that hospitals need to have mixer taps to prevent scalding. We have expressed our concerns regarding this and we have special permission to have separate hot and cold water taps. It has been explained that pregnant women are not unwell, but fit and healthy and will not overheat the tub. It is also vital that we have fast access to heating up or cooling off water if delivery is imminent. (Hyperthermia is dealt with in Appendix II). I have never known of any incidence of client scalding.

Midwifery care in labour or delivery

One issue that needs to be set up and reviewed regularly is the midwifery guidelines for practice. Setting guidelines that can act as ground rules may assist in overcoming problems at a later stage. In some units and midwifery practices, these guidelines are shared totally with parents and given to them in the form of a booklet. At Maidstone we have given out guidelines since our first waterbirths. This, we believe, means that midwives and parents both have the same starting point. I have never known of any complications where mothers do not wish to follow the guidelines. In fact I believe the opposite is true. This partnership in care again seems to reflect attitudes and values as expressed in *Changing Childbirth* (Department of Health, 1993). It may be necessary if you work in a hospital to get agreement from managers and trust approval prior to giving out hospital guidelines. Maidstone maternity unit has reviewed its guidelines every six months and in that time the fundamental attitude that prevails is a sharing of experience and partnership in care. Below I share with you a sample guideline that could be used at home or hospital. It is worth asking other colleagues, units and regional health authorities whether they have existing policies that you can utilise – in other words don't reinvent the wheel.

Guidelines for waterbirths

The midwife's clinical judgement is paramount. It is vital that the parents' previous knowledge of waterbirths is established prior to entering the water. Having discussed the use of the birthing pool, the following guidelines should be followed. In an emergency the mother needs to understand that she will be asked to leave the water.

- Criteria for mothers using the tubs:
  - There should be no known or envisaged problems.
  - Mother should be at term, i.e >37 weeks.
  - Entonox may be used in the water as pain relief. Pethidine should not have been given in the preceding three hours.
  - Induction by ARM/Prostin may use tubs, providing there are no known or envisaged problems.
  - PIH women may use the tubs for labour/delivery (B/P not > /30 above booking diastolic at onset of labour). *Evidence suggests that water lowers B/P.*
  - Previous LSCS should be referred to Senior Midwife for antenatal assessment. If the woman has had a vaginal delivery since LSCS then she may use the tub. *Risk assessment for low risk trial of scar. No evidence that intrauterine pressure altered in water.*
  - Women with ruptured membranes up to 24-36 hours may use tubs.(Apyrexial/normality) *No known risk of infection. Deep ear swab as per policy.*

- Labour should be established prior to entering water. *Once in established labour, it would appear that water enhances uterine activity.*

- Care of mother and baby as per normal practice.
  - Maternal temperature should be recorded hourly. *To prevent maternal hyperthermia.*
  - There should be ambient room temperature.
  - Fans or extractor fans should be available.

- Water temperatures:
  First stage: 33-40°C

Second stage: 37-37.5°C
Temperature should be measured and recorded every 30-60 minutes in first stage. Every 15 minutes in second stage.
Evidence suggests that this range of temperature enhances uterine activity and prevents initiation of respiration in the newborn. (Johnson 1996)

- Mother should be encouraged to drink fluids.
  To avoid dehydration in the warm environment.

- Floatation aids need to be available.

- Lifting equipment should be available if large/deep tubs used.
  Important to risk assess clinical situation. (RCN, 1996)

- Fetal auscultation should be undertaken using aqua doppler.
  To avoid any risk of electric shock/damage to the transducer.

- Water is kept as clear as possible with a sieve.
  To assist in the observation of water colour, i.e. blood or liquor.

- Care of the perineum: traditional control of the head during crowning is noted to be unnecessary. *Immersion in water appears to enhance the elasticity of the perineum. The counter pressure of the water may enable the mother to push more steadily, and thus encourage controlled delivery of the head.* (Garland & Jones, 1997)

- Suturing may be delayed for up to one hour following delivery.
  Perineal tissues may be water saturated.

- When baby is born he/she should be brought immediately to the surface. 'Baby Sam' mucus extractor available if required. *Deliver totally submerged as exposure to air will initiate respiration. Hypoxia may develop if the baby is left underwater or if the placenta starts to separate.*

- Third stage management: midwives may use discretion as to management, but no routine syntometrine given after discussion with mother. *Women need to have a labour risk assessment: Antenatal Hb level; Normal 1st and 2nd stage; No previous third stage problems; Maternal choice; Need to obtain urgent cord bloods (Abnormal fetal antibodies)* There is no evidence to support the theory of risk of water embolism.

- Estimated blood loss: Blood clots are collected using sieve EBL recorded as < or > 500 mls.
  Maternal wellbeing is assessed using clinical picture/observation.

- Emergency/abnormal situations: mother is asked to leave water.
  To reassess situation/expedite delivery.

  A resuscitaire/emergency equipment should be available in close proximity.

  Under no circumstances should the NUCHAL CORD be clamped and cut under water.

- Midwifery support for staff in training should be identified prior to the mother entering the tub.
  Second midwife only required if skill-sharing or if there is an emergency.

- Mother should be re-assessed on dry land after 5 hours.
  Evidence supports that most mothers will deliver: Primips 4-5 hours Multips 2-3 hours.

If delivery is therefore not imminent after 5 hours in the water mother should be re-assessed on dry land.

Agreement may also have to made about management of routine monitoring, free fluid policy and physiological third stage. In other words the 'fringe' issues of ground rules are as important as the actual water labour/birth guidelines.

Ten-point plan

This final ten-point plan may act as a checklist prior to starting up a hydrotherapy service.

Ten points to safe use of hydrotherapy in labour/delivery

- Clients should be low-risk and within normal criteria.
- Water temperature should be measured and recorded regularly: 1st stage 33-40°C and 2nd stage 37-37.5°C.
- Water depth should be sufficient to facilitate mobility but not deep enough to stop mother expiring her heat.
- Mother should be encouraged to drink, in order to avoid dehydration and possible hyperthermia.
- Fetal monitoring/auscultation recommended with underwater dopplers.

- Midwives should review literature and clinical advice regarding maternal and newborn physiology.
- Mother and baby should be kept warm with towels and gowns following delivery.
- Suturing may be delayed for an hour after delivery to allow tissues to revitalise.
- Midwives and parents should be encouraged to write comments about their experiences.
- Hydrotherapy appears to be a safe option for low-risk women.

Summary of principles for midwifery practice

Utilise all colleagues with particular skills and knowledge.

Find out about other midwives and units both locally and nationally that have experience with waterbirths. See Chapter Eleven for further information about midwives' education.

'Normality criteria'
- Use local and national guidelines (RCM 1997).
- Local discussion for client selection (IOL/ToS etc).
- How will women become aware of the service? Leaflets/parentcraft sessions?
- Staff education – are all staff regularly updated on theory and practice?

Antenatal preparation
- Education about waterbirthing service: parentcraft/leaflets/video. Find out how much clients already know.
- Promote the positive health aspects of aquanatal classes.
- Home birth preparation, and follow up.
- Identify birth companion, and supporter if at home. What is their knowledge of waterbirths?

Labour
- Agreed definitions of latent versus active labour.
- When to enter or leave water.
- Comfortable environment – cushions/beanbags/room thermometer and fans.

- Agreed policies on midwifery care: water temperatures/monitoring/fluids.
- CTG base tracing prior to entering pool.
- Progress of labour – agreed policy on vaginal examinations (timing and in/out of water) ARM under water.
- Emergencies... What if...?
- Completion of audit forms.
- Maintain contemporaneous records of all discussions and care during antenatal/labour/delivery and post natal period.

Delivery of newborn

- Practical versus physiological care, i.e. water depth, temperature. Use of episiotomy.
- Emergencies (consider home and hospital).

Third stage management

- Assessment of risk: woman's general health; Hb; previous third stage problems; non-intervention labour; nature of contractions; first and second stage; newborn size; need to obtain cord bloods; and maternal choice.
- Physiological versus active management (consider midwives' skills: in water versus out of water).
- Post-natal care.
- Midwifery care and observations. Are local policies agreed on newborn observations (see Forde *et al*, 1999)?
- Suturing – this may need to be delayed (waiting for placenta to deliver and perineal tissue to revitalise after waterbirth).
- Promotion of breast feeding – to assist physiological third stage and skin to skin contact/warmth for baby.

(Cited Milner 1988, Ford and Garland 1989)

CHAPTER SIX

Positive health aspects of hydrotherapy

Swimming has long been known as an enjoyable and strong relaxant. It is something that every member of the family can benefit from and it is a form of exercise that can bestow positive health aspects. Water can be used by all age groups and it is well known that it can be used by even the most compromised individual. Exercise in water can, therefore, be the most beneficial form of exercise for expectant mothers and one that can be extended into the postnatal period.

As midwives, we aim to promote physical and mental wellbeing in women during their pregnancies. They are encouraged not to smoke or drink, to attend antenatal classes to learn about what will happen to their bodies and prepare themselves physically and mentally for labour. The physical effort of labour and delivery has been likened to running a marathon. How many women really undertake the training programme to plan for the labour? We somehow expect that pregnant women can undertake these rigours without adequate preparation. No athlete would do a marathon without weeks and months of planning. As midwives we have nine months with which to plan with our mothers for the work ahead.

Finding an organised class

Many local swimming pools have started aquanatal classes and it is worth searching local papers to see what is available. Since about 1987 the National Sports Stadium at Crystal Palace, London, have been undertaking organised antenatal swimming. They are professionally organised and run by trained staff who have gone through the aquafit course. It is important that those taking the class have the correct qualifications. As midwives, if we wish to run similar classes, it is worth investigating local training courses and reviewing your Code of Practice with regard to acquiring new skills.

Midwives who take aquanatal swimming should ensure that they are adequately trained in other skills as well as aquafit. You may need to have life-saving skills, especially if the local pool does not provide a female life saver. Midwives also need to have an ability to organise and have some idea of rhythm (golden oldies appear to play well in pool acoustics!).

When actually taking the classes, it is beneficial to have one midwife in the pool and one outside demonstrating. It's worth tying back long hair, wearing no distracting jewellery and having a well-fitting sports bra and costume. You should have up-to-date information for the women with possibly handouts. You will need access to a cassette player and a variety of flotation aids.

Administration of aquafit classes

Pool
A graduated pool allows for greater flexibility of classes. The shallow end encourages non-swimmers to join in and facilitates a relaxation area between exercises. In the shallow end it is easier to undertake partner work and a greater variety of exercises. In the deep end women are encouraged to work against the increased water pressure. The deep end is also better and more comfortable for taller women. A graduated pool is more useful and allows circuit-training to take place. Access should be via stairs and not a ladder.

Water temperature
Warm water at 28-30°C appears to reduce tension and relax muscles. If the water is too cool, antenatal women may get muscle cramps. In water that is too hot, the women may feel dizzy and lethargic.

Changing room
The women need privacy, they usually prefer individual cubicles and not communal areas. It is also important that the women have space to wheel in prams, if a postnatal class is also run.

Pool use

It is preferred that the pool is used exclusively by these women but this usually costs more. Exclusive use appears to be more relaxing, privacy is ensured and opens the classes to all groups (Asian and Jewish women). It is worth remembering that in an ordinary pool, the noise of excited children swimming can be very disturbing and distract from the teacher running the class.

The cost of pool hire should be investigated. Is it cheaper to hire the pool and split the cost between women, or allow the pool to hire out and charge to women direct? In our experience we have found the best avenue is to self-hire and divide the cost of hire between the women. Any profits can be used to pay for courses and equipment.

You will need to check fire drills and exits. Insurance in the pool will need to be checked. You may need to get public liability insurance or your vicarious liability, if employed by the NHS, may cover your practice. If you are a Royal College of Midwives member and you are undertaking midwifery duties for which you are trained, then your insurance will cover you regardless of being on duty or not. It is worth checking with your local supervisor of midwives regarding your role. A final note of caution is that if you are undertaking this outside your normal working hours you should be aware that many Trusts have clauses which forbid you undertaking services that are in direct competition with the Trust.

Advertising

You can advertise in local newspapers, on hospital and community notice boards and anywhere that pregnant women go! It's also worthwhile trying a spot on local radio or television. We have found that word of mouth is both the best way of advertising and promoting the service. At first you may need to survey women locally to check there is a demand for this service.

Mothers' preparation

We give out a questionnaire to all women prior to attending the class; a sample is shown in Table 6.1. If in any doubt they are always asked to seek medical approval first. We advise our ladies to wear a sports bra or maternity swimsuit (or extra large T-shirt). Tying long hair back and taking off jewellery all assist in ease of exercise. Women may wish to have a drink available on the side of the pool.

Table 6.1: Sample questionnaire

Have you experienced any of these problems during this pregnancy:

- threatened miscarriage
- bleeding
- raised blood pressure
- recurrent infections, i.e. urine
- baby not growing.

Women are advised that after the session they should have a shower and apply a lotion or moisturiser. It's important that the women give themselves time to unwind and relax with a drink for about 20 minutes after the session.

It almost goes without saying but the session should be fun, otherwise the women will not return. The aim of aquafit is for the women to enter labour in the optimum condition, healthy and as fit as possible. Other authors who have written about setting up aquanatal classes include Halksworth (1994), Cain (1992) and Baddeley (1993).

Having arranged yourself and the pool it's now time to start the exercises and relaxation. Water acts as a veil for pregnant women. They can lose many of their inhibitions in water and many women actually feel elegant for the first time in months. This attitude to offering a relaxed atmosphere for pregnant women was described by Oudshoorn (1990) when she writes about the situation in The Netherlands. The classes consist of exercises and a type of water 'ballet'. Water aids buoyancy and reduces energy expenditure, both of which are useful to a heavily pregnant woman.

Exercises in water allow the woman to exercise against the pressure of the water and enhance muscle activity. It is easy to utilise all muscles and work them through a full range of movement. Because of the buoyancy in water, support is offered to the women making the chance of strains and stress less likely. The body should be almost completely immersed, as this encourages movement and keeps the mother in a warm environment. Minor aches and pains can be eased greatly by warm water; backache, in particular, seems to be eased in this environment.

Physiological benefits of aquafit

Aquafit is one of the best all round exercises to take part in during pregnancy. It is excellent at building up stamina, strength and suppleness in an environment that does not place extra strain on the woman's body. The feeling of weightlessness allows the woman to move her joints more freely and with less effort than on dry land. Combined with the effects of heat, buoyancy enables a greater range of movements to be achieved. Exercise in water has well-documented physiological benefits. Skinner and Thomson (1986) write:

> water acts as a pain relief and reduces muscle spasm, strengthening of muscles and developing their power and endurance, increases circulation and improving client morale.

Physiological changes occur to every part of the woman's body and water exercise can enhance blood supply to the heart and lungs. Increased relaxation gives a sense of wellbeing with the release of nature's pain killers, endorphins. The relaxation qualities of water mean that when the woman is submerged, with only the head and neck out, she can gain a 90 per cent reduction in body weight. Considering the fact that most women put on approximately 12kg in pregnancy, this reduction has obvious benefits. Relaxation is also a time for the women to come into focus with her body and baby. Many experience such a degree of relaxation that they actually fall asleep in the water. The local classes that I have visited show that it is often necessary to ask midwives to be in the pool at this time to stop the women 'bumping' into each other.

Changes to the cardiovascular system and its effect in aquafit

The changes to a pregnant woman include a 50 per cent increase in plasma volume, 40 per cent cardiac output, slight fall in blood pressure in second trimester and a fall in peripheral resistance. It has been documented that aquanatal swimming does not cause any significant changes. It is worth reviewing physiological benefits in labour (Chapter Seven) where it is stated that blood pressure reduces with hydrotherapy.

Renal changes

The glomerular filtration rate increases by 40-60 per cent and plasma flow increases. There may be effects in water but these tend to be short-lived. There appear to be no reported negative effects to mother or baby when using aquafit.

When should a woman start exercising?

Unless there are any complications with the pregnancy, it is good to start exercising as soon as possible. The more exercise a pregnant woman takes the better she feels and looks. It will keep her in good shape and prepare her for the labour and delivery ahead. I do not believe that aquanatal swimming is a prerequisite to water labour/delivery but the 'flotation sensation' experienced by women can take a little getting used to.

Does water exercise shorten labour?

Ketter and Shelton (1984) write that it has not been proved that labour is shorter or less painful if the women has used aquafit. Women who do exercise express positive thoughts about themselves and often feel well prepared for labour and delivery. In Chapter Seven the benefits of relaxation on hormonal balance are shown. A relaxed woman can ease her own labour and delivery by feeling more in control.

The exercise programme

Although most aquafit classes are run by experienced teachers, many women find that they can follow through the programme on their own at other times during the week. The basic principle is to remember to use the water for its buoyancy and negative gravity effects. This means asking mothers to stay as submerged as possible during the programme. All exercise programmes are based around a warming-up period, exercises (both physical and mental) and a slowing down relaxing session. Several good books have been written about aquafit (Hughes, 1989). They should be reviewed by anyone wishing to start these exercise programmes.

Summarised advantages of aquafit classes

- Social event for expectant women and mothers with newborn babies.
- Women feel more graceful and 'weightless', enhancing self-esteem.
- Freedom of movement in water.
- Exercise is available to most women and is not dependent upon previous exercise history.
- Water is environmentally friendly and babies seem to like it!
- Certain exercises are easier to perform in water where resistance is greater.

- Water places minimal strain on joints and ligaments.
- All body systems can be stimulated in a safe environment.

One author who has written widely on the subject of aquanatal classes is Baddeley. In a paper presented in ICM Manila 1999 she continued her work on the advantages of using water for exercising, exploring both the physical and psychological benefits.

Postnatal exercises

Many mothers, having experienced antenatal swimming, wish to continue with this exercise postnatally. I usually advise mothers to wait for their six-week postnatal appointment before recommencing and for those who have had a caesarean section a medical opinion may be valid. A rule of thumb is that six weeks seem to be the best time to start (or when bleeding stops) so long as there are no known or envisaged complications.

Many classes run with antenatal and postnatal sessions. Our classes start with the postnatal mothers and then an antenatal session. This provides a good opportunity for new mothers to meet each other and for expectant mothers to see newborn babies (perhaps for the first time).

The type of exercises alter postnatally, as we now concentrate on thighs and waistlines. It is worth recommending that mothers exercise for at least three months postnatally, although I hope they will continue for life. Mother and baby classes are often run by local swimming pools, usually these commence after the first vaccinations (Farnworth, 1990).

Mother and baby classes

Many swimming pools run classes designed for mothers and babies, giving them the privacy and private sessions that they require. Whilst it may be outside the remit of midwives to get actively involved, our health visitor colleagues may well find another avenue for social and professional contact. It is an ideal opportunity to meet new mothers and provides an insight into mother and baby interaction. We can watch as the family develops and assess any areas of parenting skills that may need enhancing. Newborns generally appear to enjoy the water play and as Freud wrote, 'Never underestimate the importance of play'. Pattison (1996) writes about the benefits to both mother and baby during the antenatal and postnatal period.

Disadvantages and contraindications of aquafit

The initial start-up costs of aquafit may be high and you should consider the ongoing costs of insurance and pool cost increases. There are few contraindications to using water in pregnancy or the postnatal period. Generally it is worth ensuring that no one using the pool has an infection. That includes the midwives attending the session. As already stated, if the woman has any medical or obstetrical complications, it is worth checking with a doctor prior to commencing aquafit.

In our experience there has never been an accident at the pool with either mothers, babies or midwives. The women using the pool are fit and healthy and are no more likely to slip than at any other time. If an untoward incident does occur, it is worth finding out what local pool guidelines exist.

Conclusion

This summary of an aquafit action plan may assist you in planning your course.

Points to consider:

- **The pool**
  Pool hire
  Pool depth (graduated is best)
  Water temperature (28°C–30°C).
- **Midwife training**
  ASA/Aquafit
  Lifesaver skills
  Ability to organise
  Must have rhythm!
  At least two midwives at the pool – one in water and one on the poolside.
- **Insurance**
  Vicarious or public liability.
- **Advertising**
  Through local schools, surgeries, radio and papers
  Word of mouth.
- **Equipment**
  Flotation aids
  Battery-operated cassette player.

- Creche facilities.
- Private changing facilities/exclusive pool hire.
- Survey of women – service demand.
- Prerequisite for water labour/birth.
- Enthusiasm and ability to make it fun!
- See Appendix VI for aquarobics addresses.

CHAPTER SEVEN

Maternal perspective on using water in labour and delivery

Why do mothers choose a water labour or birth? Many reasons have been postulated, from a quiet, private and comforting environment to encouraging the woman to regain control of her labour. I think the answer is much simpler. Where would you go at the end of a long hard day at work, with every muscle aching and a need to escape from your family, children and home! Compound this with dysmenorrhagia, and many women say they would head for a hot bath, with a long cool drink! Is it therefore surprising that this situation is remembered by women in labour, who 'naturally' head for water?

Think carefully about this scenario, as I share with you the physiological and psychological benefits of using water in labour and delivery. Remember that using water as an early labour relaxant is not new. How many of us grew up professionally with the idea of steering women to a bathtub before they come into hospital. If we are to explore the advantages of water, it's worth reviewing the normal changes to a woman's body during the course of labour.

Physiology of pain and reactions to labour

When a woman goes into labour, however well-prepared physically and mentally she is, her body will undergo major changes. These can be identified as stress, pain, reduced mobility and fatigue. As midwives, we aim to prepare women for these changes through antenatal preparation programmes and education. As long ago as 1920, Grantly Dick-Read identified a cycle of interplay between these factors and labour outcome.

However well-prepared the woman is for labour, the nature of her pain is also dependent upon previous experiences, her own pain perception and tolerance threshold. Moore (1994) wrote about pain relief in labour from both a historical view and its present-day management.

Stress in labour

Why does stress play such a part in the way that labour progresses? What is stress? It's a reaction to a particular situation, in some cases being helpful, in others a hindrance. Stress is caused by several factors, psychologically through fear, worry, anxiety and anger. Physically, stress occurs when there is an injury or illness, in the presence of pain or hypoxia. All these areas could be relevant in labour and I suspect we can all think of ways we aim to reduce these stress levels.

Can some 'stressors' actually be beneficial to women in labour? As they are a reaction to a specific situation, could they assist in promoting or adapting a homeostasis? Could these stressors play a part in the fine interplay that appears to exist between a woman's physiological and psychological state of wellbeing? Can they facilitate a return to the normal balance in her body? I would suggest that in many cases the answer is positive. Women appear to have an amazing ability to cope with labour and delivery. As we expand our horizons in what is thought to be 'normal' labour, we realise that the parameters set in the past for a one-hour second stage for a primigravida may well not be relevant (Crawford, 1987). Every woman is an individual and, as such, her labour, ability to cope with that labour and delivery is individual.

This issue of normal labour physiology was reviewed by Odent (1997) especially when a woman enters the water pool early in labour. The fine interplay of hormonal influences during labour, particularly atrial natriuretic peptide, and its ultimate effect via the posterior pituitary gland on oxytocins has, Odent stated, been poorly studied.

Odent suggests that water should be available and, indeed, anticipated for use in labour. He believes water temperature should not exceed 37°C (although many practitioners would agree differently, providing that adequate guidelines are given) and the measurement of the efficiency of water as a pain relief, after two hours immersion.

However, I do believe that as midwives we should encourage wider individuality in our care, and that if we limit each woman's time spent in the water, according to centimetres dilated and water temperature then she is not seen as a unique individual.

This individuality is, I suspect, why we see such varying labours. As in some women these stressors act positively whilst in others they provoke a negative reaction. Whether they cause a positive or negative reaction depends, I believe, on the woman's own adaptability as a person.

Normal adaptive process (NAP)

During labour the fine interplay of hormones rise as labour progresses. This interplay exists between catecholamines, adrenaline and noradrenaline and the normal hormones of labour, oxytocin and endorphins. The normal rise in hormones can be seen in Fig. 7.1. They increase with fear and anxiety and may actually become harmful when excessive levels are reached. In this situation there may be a possible shunting of blood flow away from the uterine circulation.

The NAP is a normal reaction that is said to assist the fetus in his preparation for extrauterine life. This process with its hormonal response:

- promotes absorption of lung fluid
- protects the heart and brain against hypoxia
- assists the baby to maintain his body temperature.

Can this be related to clinical practice? How often have we as midwives been confronted with apparent signs of 'fetal distress', which at delivery is not borne out by the Apgar scores and is unrelated to signs of neonatal problems? This is not to say that we should be complacent regarding fetal distress but just as I have said that each mother should be treated as an individual so too should the baby. Many will cope with the rigours of labour and delivery without any signs of compromise, whilst others will react very quickly to changes in his intrauterine environment. How dependent the baby is on mother's physical and psychological wellbeing can be reviewed in Appendix I.

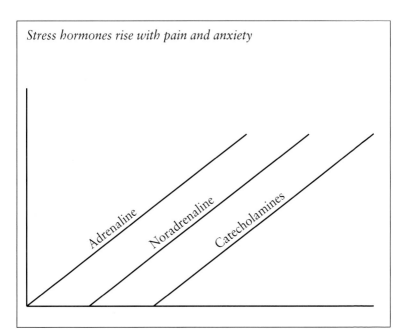

Fig. 7.1: Normal adaptive process

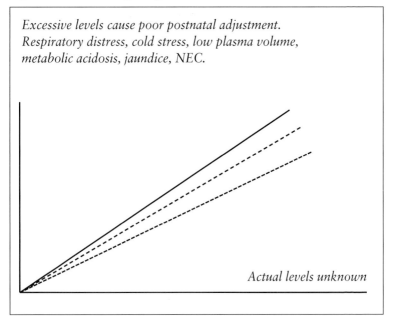

Fig. 7.2: Postnatal period

Pain in labour

What causes the pain of labour? Pain results from intense stimuli, which may cause or threaten to cause tissue damage. The pain receptors respond to this stimuli and assist in avoiding or minimizing bodily damage. We know that if pain occurs during labour then there is a rise in catecholamines and corticosteriods, with a potential to cause maternal acidosis and a reduction in uterine activity.

Reduced mobility in labour

The reduction in mobility in labour is caused by two issues. The first is that it becomes increasingly difficult to mobilise when on dry land and secondly, our modern day beds and monitoring equipment do not always lend themselves to mobility. Some efforts have been made with the introduction of birthing stools and beds and telemetry monitoring but that still does not overcome the problem of a heavily pregnant woman physically moving herself during labour. This reduction in mobility causes potential for vena caval compression and the inherent risk of maternal hypotension and reduced placental blood flow.

Fatigue in labour

As labour commences the woman will experience a degree of reduced gastrointestinal absorption and dehydration as gastric emptying is slowed and reserves are utilised in labour. This may be compounded where the woman is unable or prevented from eating and drinking. Many units still practice in an environment that does not encourage labouring women (low-risk) to eat and drink. Much has been written about providing a neutral gastric contents situation, with the recommendation of an oral preparation, i.e. Ranitidine.

Having considered these four areas of normal physiology, it is worth exploring the effects of hormones in labour. Fig. 7.3 is a summary of what other authors have written about the hormonal interplay. Full details are given in the Reference List at the end of the book.

Adrenaline – the so-called fight and flight hormone

- Increased levels occur with fear and cold (Odent, 1981).
- Increased levels can inhibit labour (Lenstrup, 1987).
- Adrenaline is said to trigger the fetus ejection reflex (Odent, 1987).
- Studies on ewes showed that noradrenaline may cause cardiovascular changes (Falconer, 1982).

Catecholamines

- Normal amounts may help the fetus to withstand oxygen deprivation in labour (Simkin, 1990).

- Excessive levels (through stress) may cause dysfunctional labour, decreased uterine tone, slower dilation and resulting hypoxia (Simkin, 1990).

- Fetus ejection reflex occurs with increased levels (Odent, 1987).

- Appear to have increased levels with progressive cervical dilation (Falconer, 1982).

Endorphins

- Endorphins suppress smooth muscle, relieve pain, enhance memory mechanisms, cause euphoria; regulate other hormones, such as growth hormone, gonadotrophic releasing hormone, oestrogen and oxytocin.

- Optimal levels are reached during altered conscious state (Odent, 1981).

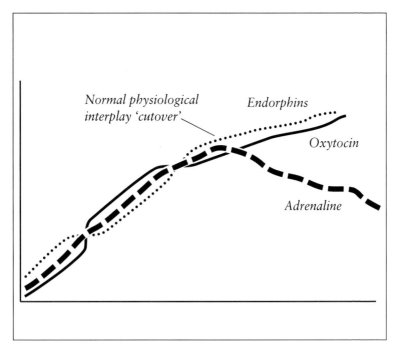

Fig. 7.3: Hormonal interplay

• Normal endorphins are inhibited and suppressed by adrenaline (Milner, 1988).

Oxytocin

Optimal levels occur with altered conscious state (Odent, 1981).

Cortisol

High levels may suppress fetal ACTH production and thereby oestriol synthesis (Maltau, 1979).

Throughout labour and with the attitude to care that we plan, our aim is to reduce the production of catecholamines and other stress-related hormones. There are two ways to alter the hormonal balance:

Medical model	Midwifery model
Active management of labour	Non-intervention
Hormonal infusions	Support with Dhoulas
High use of technology	Complementary therapies
	Comfortable environment

As midwives we are aiming to provide a safe and supportive environment within which to care for women. Even by just reviewing our use of technology with a more judicious attitude we may well alter patterns of care. So can we use all this physiological knowledge in our midwifery practice? The basic difference between obstetricians and midwives is more than the difference in training. Even our two titles bear the hallmarks of two different professions. Obstetrician is derived from the Latin – Obsto – I stand in front (interestingly the word obstacle comes from the same route). Midwife, on the other hand means, with woman. Maybe this fundamental issue can shed light upon why our two professions have grown up so differently. Brook (1976) writing about midwives states:

> Midwives' work was based on belief in the evidence of the senses. She trusted, and the pregnant woman trusted in her, to find ways to deal with the hazards of pregnancy and childbirth.

He continues (pp. 41-42):

> that midwives were viewed as witches as it was claimed they had magical powers... simply because they were well-versed in the healing properties of herbs and used them medically.

Benefits of water compared to other pain relief

TENS

The woman is in control of this pain relief, she is aware of her surroundings, can remain mobile and is drug free. She may have to use a hired unit, if not available in the hospital or community setting. TENS (Transcutaneous Electrical Nerve Stimulation) can be used with other forms of pain relief except water. There have been few reported incidences of interference with electronic monitoring. Physiological properties are based on 'gate control theory' (Melzack *et al*, 1965).

Entonox

With its combination of oxygen and nitrous oxide, this is a low solubility drug. It is utilised through the lung and arterial blood stream. Only relatively small amounts are required to saturate blood, thus high levels of arterial and brain tension of drug. Disadvantages include the need to start inhalation at the beginning of contractions and thus there is a timing issue. Some mothers do not like the mask or the mouthpiece and gas may make mothers feel nauseous. It is used by 60 per cent of women in labour.

Meptazinol

This is a non-narcotic analgesia, used for the treatment of moderate to severe pain. Few side effects have been recorded. Its disadvantages are that it may cause nausea, drowsiness and dizziness. Mild effects on the fetus can be in part be reversed by Naloxone. Meptazinol is used by 1.8 per cent of women in labour.

Pethidine

Acts on opiate receptors at the neurone, causing analgesia, euphoria, sedation and possibly respiratory depression. The disadvantages include nausea and placental cross-over to the fetus. Used by 37 per cent of women in labour.

Epidural

Marcaine in epidural block infiltrates the small diameter autonomic nerve fibres thus blocking them. Has advantage of slow onset – long duration (Neal, 1987). Disadvantages of epidural stem from the change to the potential physiology of labour. Changes to blood pressure could cause compromise to the baby. Reports have been shown that some women suffer long-term sequelae with backache. Used by 18 per cent of women in labour.

Physiological benefits of hydrotherapy

So how does water work, what properties does it possess that makes it an option that women wish for in labour? Some would say that is simply that water is relaxing in a pleasant environment and undertaken by caring people (Stanway, 1979). Others say that water properties are not dissimilar to TENS with the gate control theory, endogenous pain control theory and as a distraction therapy (Brucker, 1984). The physiological properties have been known for many years with studies undertaken as early as 1847, cited by Goodlin *et al* (1984), where the diuretic and haemodynamic qualities are discussed.

Changes have been reported in core temperature in water over 35°C. Whether this is significant or not may depend on other factors as explained in Appendix II. A study by Weston *et al* (1987) also showed an increase in cardiac index and stroke volume. They continue by stating that the major effects are haemodynamic and renal and although their study was not completed on pregnant women we should be aware of these issues. In studies by Katz *et al* (1988) immersion in water did not cause any elevation in temperature or heart rate, although the fetuses on ultrasound were found to be in an active state.

It is not possible in this book to write the full details of the benefits of using water – that would be a text all of its own. Below are summaries of the physiological, psychological and pathological benefits of water with references to some of the theories given at the end of the chapter if you wish to follow them up.

Summary of physiological benefits
- Increases relaxation
- Decreases pain
- Decreases pressure on abdominal muscles and vena cava
- Increases pelvic diameters
- Increases buoyancy and mobility
- Gravity-free environment
- Increases contractions
- Increases endorphin and oxytocin production
- Increases oxygen and blood supply
- Increases peripheral/muscle and skin temperature
- Increases velocity of nerve conduction
- Increases tissue metabolism

- Relaxes perineal tissue
- Reduces blood pressure

Summary of psychological benefits
- Flotation sensation
- Increases experience of pregnancy, labour and delivery
- Increases self-control
- Decreases fear and anger
- Increases self-awareness and consciousness during labour and delivery
- Increases pain threshold
- Secure, warm, private and quiet environment
- Pleasurable, reassuring and serene effect
- Increases receptiveness to baby
- Increases mother and baby interaction
- Symbolic relationship
- Increases emotional experience for care giver

Summary of pathological benefits
- Reduces blood pressure
- Increases diuresis and removal of other waste products
- Reduces noradrenaline and adrenaline
- Reduces sensory stimulation
- Reduces pain perception
- Reduces use of other analgesics
- Reduces use of augmentation

Many women have written about their personal experiences and, as one might expect, they provide an enthusiastic and vivid description of waterbirth. The benefits and advantages may be described as twofold – control over labour and delivery and a feeling of general wellbeing. Whether these advantages have any long-term effect on maternal-newborn bonding or long-term child development have yet to be shown. From personal experience I would say that waterbirth does have a positive effect on the woman's perception of her birth. The words used to describe their delivery are calmness and peaceful, not the usual words one hears. Many do breastfeed and feel physically and psychologically well prepared to take on this role. They do not feel exhausted after delivery and many say they could actually go through delivery again the next day! (See Chapter Eleven.)

Conclusion

The relative benefits of using water for labour and delivery have yet to be fully explored and perhaps researched. It is true that many of the positive aspects are subjective but in a consumer-led service and at a time when women are regaining control, it would seem paramount that we aim to provide this type of care. Many advantages are being studied, and not always in our own discipline so it is therefore important that we network and learn from other professionals.

CHAPTER EIGHT

Fetal and newborn perspective

One of the most contentious subjects currently under discussion is abortion. The anti-abortionist lobby state that as the soul enters the fetus at conception, he or she thus has an entity of his or her own from day one. When does the soul enter the fetus and when does that make a mother aware that the baby has a life of its own?

Wambach (1979) attempted to answer some of these questions in her book. A study group of 750 people were put under hypnosis and asked to recall their memories of in utero life, labour and delivery. This book is fascinating to read and appears to purport the theory that the baby is a separate entity early in utero and certainly by six months.

Many women have stated that their attachment towards their baby started when they felt the fetus move or towards the time when the baby was due. Has this attachment changed in light of today's current midwifery practice? We stress to mothers the importance of diet and avoidance of certain substances. Ultrasound scans have revolutionised the way that mothers now perceive their unborn baby – to see the fetus from ten weeks and watch him develop over the next few months must be fantastic. Has this increased awareness improved our perception of his needs?

How, as midwives, can we improve our care at the time of birth and utilise this knowledge? Are we aware that hearing is the most finely developed sense in utero? Can we ensure that the baby is delivered into a quiet room, keeping noise to a minimum? We can reduce stimuli by dimming the lights and keeping mother and baby together with skin-to-skin contact for as long as possible. This skin-to-skin contact was studied by Klaus and Kennell (1982). 'Routine' procedures such as bathing and weighing should be left as long as possible to enable the baby to familiarise himself with the outside world. This theme is further suggested by Morris (1991). We should be promote early feeding in the first few hours after birth, which has been shown to improve breastfeeding success (Salariya, Easton and Cater, 1978).

We are also more aware of the fine interplay that exists between mother and baby. We stress to mothers the importance of avoiding certain substances during pregnancy and that infections and cigarettes can have a profound effect on fetal development. Could this fine interplay become so overwhelming that it actually places the baby in a vulnerable position? (See Appendix I.)

Verny (1987) appears to agree with other authors that this fine interplay between mother and baby causes all her insecurities and anxieties to be relayed to the baby. Continual or intense anxiety, and thus an increase in hormones, could cause hazards to him. Assaults on the baby from smoking and drinking all have an effect, when what he really wants is love and attention and a chance to bond with his mother. Verny continues that at this vulnerable stage of birth the bombardment of stimuli triggers respiration and the first cry. Is that cry of joy or a way of communicating distress and subsequently his needs? He writes, (p.86):

Even in the best circumstances, birth reverberates through the child's body like a seismic shock of earthquake proportions.

Even though the oxytocin produced in labour is said to be an amnesiac, nothing, according to Verny, will escape the baby's memory, every feeling, every movement is remembered. The study undertaken by Wambach studied 750 people who, under hypnosis regressed to their own labours and deliveries. The work reported some interesting thoughts by these subjects. Many are quoted as saying that they found their births a time of great sadness and that on emerging from the womb:

they reported a rush of physical sensations... that was disturbing and unpleasant (p.122).

Wambach continues that this was expressed by the subjects as a hesitancy at being born. Can this knowledge be utilised today, could we as midwives identify with this in our modern day labour rooms? How often have you discussed the possibility of forceps with a woman, who is having a slow second stage, and suddenly find her delivering with the next few contractions? Could this be an explanation to Odent's 'fetus ejection reflex'? Wambach continues:

> the physical senses (having) so much vivid input that the soul feels almost 'drowned' in light, cold air and sounds.

Development of newborns

In utero babies are subjected to increasing amounts of circulating hormones that promote development and growth. Crossover of adrenal steroids via the placenta is said by Pearce (1977) to leave the fetus and infant 'locked in a free floating anxiety'.

Stress hormones are 20 times higher in a baby than an adult and ten times higher in a mother giving birth. This increase in hormone levels and the inherent 'normal' physiological hypoxia of labour is usually transient. We are aware as midwives that this process is counteracted by the fetal haemoglobin (fHb) properties and its high circulating level. Stress hormones, i.e. catecholamines, counteract the effects of oxygen deprivation by increasing blood pressure and heart output, especially to vital organs. This birth stress is due, in part, to the circulating hormones but also to the physical passage of birth with all its inherent trauma and hazards. The arousal state that the newborn baby exerts at delivery, heightened by its bonding with mother shows as an alertness of the baby's body and brain as written by Pearce.

This theme is continued by Balaskas and Gordon (1990) reminding us that babies are well adapted for the stresses of labour and delivery. The physiological contraction and relaxation of uterine muscle enables the baby to cope with the described physiological oxygen deprivation.

Effects of drugs on the fetus and newborn

In labour, most forms of pain relief could potentially have an effect on the fetus and on the baby once delivered. The advantages and disadvantages of each needs to be considered by mother and midwife prior to administration. The introduction of non-invasive forms of pain relief, i.e. Transcutaneous Electrical Nerve Stimulation (TENS) has given more choice to women. Other forms of pain relief more currently used are Pethidine and Epidural. Pethidine is well-documented as potentially causing drowsiness and unresponsive babies at delivery (Brook, 1976), producing reduced sucking and lowered maternal interaction following delivery. It is stated that a baby in utero receives 20 times the maternal dose of Pethidine and, not surprisingly therefore, that it has been measured in newborns' blood up to seven days postnatally. Brook continues by saying:

> The onus is on the medical profession to prove that a pharmacological labour is superior.

It is within these parameters that water labour and birth has become fashionable. As already stated, the true background and history may never be proved. It is therefore up to those professionals undertaking this therapy to show that it is truly a safe option for labour and delivery.

Fetal perspective on waterbirth

Waterbirths have been introduced in many units at a time when medical intervention has peaked. The attitudes towards maternal and fetal interplay have shown very clearly that the two cannot be separated. Mothers' early awareness of their babies has lent itself towards a non-interventionist attitude to care. Midwives have attempted to make delivery rooms as 'user friendly' as possible, with 'home-like birthing rooms'. We may never manage the luxury of American birthing centres (Fig. 8.1) but the traditional labour room may well be a thing of the past. Even before 'Winterton' and *Changing Childbirth*, reports had spurned the traditional way of routine procedures (shaves and enemas) and non-personalised attitude to care.

There are many fringe issues surrounding the introduction of waterbirth (see Chapter One) and these may need to be addressed prior to water being a feasible option for your unit. Leboyer (p.5, 1974) wrote:

> The simple fact is that as soon as a child is born he starts to cry and how bitterly. And although this is strange, it is the one thing that delights everyone there... how beautifully my child cries exclaims the happy mother, thrilled and amazed that something so little can make so much noise.

This quote written 20 years ago seems to have as much relevance in today's society as when it was written. Does crying simply mean that all

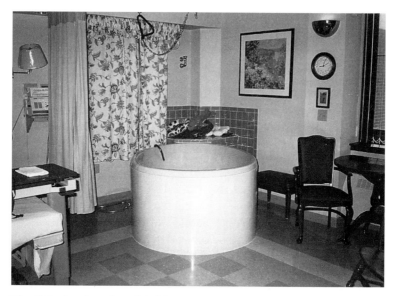

Fig. 8.1: An American birthing centre

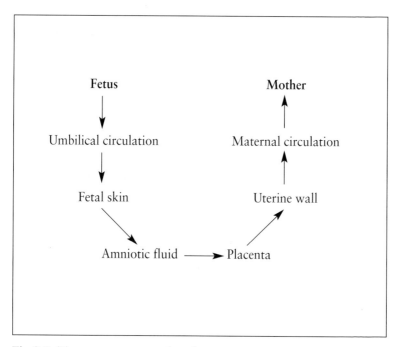

Fig 8.2: Temperature control pathway

the baby's reflexes and senses are working? Or is the baby trying to express something else – pain, suffering or sorrow? Leboyer's work was twofold, not to cause the baby unnecessary distress and to make the newborn as comfortable as possible by welcoming him or her into the world with a bath in warm water.

Morris (1991) continues with this theme by stating that crying may be a sign of distress and baby panic – not as parents feel, a joyous arrival of their baby, and for midwives, the stimulation for respiration.

Through the baby's senses we can explore the environment of the fetus. In 1909 Giles wrote (cited *Brave New Babies*, Channel 4):

The senses lie dormant when the child is in the womb: in the darkness and quiet of its aquatic existence it sees nothing, hears nothing; it neither tastes nor smells; no variations of temperature occur to stimulate it and even the sense of touch is hardly called into play because the fluid, in which it lies presses on it evenly and without variation.

We once thought that babies could not see in utero but we now realise that he is aware of light sensations through the uterine wall. So we have learnt to dim our lights in labour rooms and remove the bright spot light at delivery. The baby is aware of noises, he can hear his mother's voice and the loudest sound, her heartbeat. He is in a muffled world but they are the sounds of his world, which we can mimic at birth. Can we learn from this in utero environment? Leboyer (1974) believes we can:

We were wondering about how best to prepare the child... now we see it's not the child who needs to be prepared. It is ourselves. It is our eyes that need to be open, our blindness that has to stop. If we used just a little intelligence how simple things could be. (p.45)

I have mentioned several factors that can alter the mother and baby perception at birth. Could we use this knowledge to reduce stress levels and enhance the birth experience? Modern birth has not 'relaxed' our mothers – giving birth in hospitals in unfamiliar places, with unfamiliar people causes stress and anxiety. This in turn could increase hormonal output, lengthen labour and the use of interventions and thus in turn increase the level of stress on the baby. This balance of hormones may well work in other directions. How many times have you heard of couples, desperate to have a baby, who have given up all hope only to find themselves pregnant!

America's 'Rebirthing' phenomenon was a way of paving the way for future generations. By reliving our birthing experience, it is thought that we are more aware of how to pave the way for our own deliveries and that this is a life-long link.

In the 1960s Tjarkovsky originated a concept that has been explored in Russia. He felt that waterbirth was a gradual introduction to the world, reducing gravitational pull at delivery and assisting in reducing oxygen requirements. You may wish to read about Tjarkovsky's work in Napierala (1994). Although unsubstantiated, it is a theme continued by Ray (1986). She writes that the increase in energy required at birth can be neutralised in a gravity-free environment.

We can delve deeper into history to see the original concepts of water. In Odent's book *Entering the World* (1984), he refers back to the 14th century when a monk, Bartholomew, who was a predecessor to Leboyer, advocated a warm bath and dark place to sleep for newborn babies. Gradually we have attempted to heed these words and advocate a gentle and delicate birth. Montessori in the 20th century spoke about our apparent disregard for the delicacy of a baby at birth.

So is water a familiar environment, one which offers a baby a soothing and peaceful delivery? Balaskas and Gordon (1990) write that water reduces sensory stimulation at the time of birth and provides a loving and sensitive welcome into the world. Morris (1991, p.117) continues this theme by writing:

> *The newborn emerges into very warm water, an environment that is much closer to that in the womb. This enables it to take on it's new challenges one at a time instead of explosively, all at once.*

Finally, Lichy and Herzburg (1993) conclude by writing:

> *I want mothers to be in the best possible condition to greet and bond with their newborn babies.*

Their experiences have shown that babies born in water are often sleepy and quiet, perhaps due to the gentle transition from womb to world or because the mother has feelings of peace and tranquillity. Water is a strong relaxant for mothers – does it have a similar effect on babies? Just how aware are they of their internal and external environment? Two issues, therefore, need to be explored by care givers prior to undertaking waterbirth. First, I shall address the area of fetal heat adaptation and secondly, the extrauterine stimuli to respiration.

Fetal heat adaptation

The fetus is very dependent on his mother for heat transfer. Temperature control is based on heat transfer via a pathway between mother and baby as shown in Figure 8.2 (cited Power, 1989).

The placenta acts as a heat exchanger between mother and baby which assists in maintaining the fetal temperature 0.5-1°C above the mother's. This balance of heat control is dependent upon the temperature of the surrounding maternal tissues. At birth, the newborn thermal regulation is poor, the baby has reduced subcutaneous layers of fat and heat loss is said to be four times higher than the adult. Heat loss through evaporation is reduced in the presence of vernix and the fine thermal control can be further affected by hypoxia and hypoglycaemia. The effects of cold on the newborn, with temperatures between 27°C and 32°C in the presence of hypoglycaemia, can cause a higher incidence of pulmonary haemorrhage. For clinical practice these issues need to be addressed with the availability of warm towels for the baby and drying excess water off after delivery.

Fetal protection against inhaling water

In April 1995 the first international conference on waterbirths was held at Wembley, London. During the conference Dr Paul Johnson (physiologist at John Radcliffe Hospital, Oxford) presented a short paper highlighting why he believes babies are well adapted, indeed protected, for waterbirth. He said, 'Some things are in favour of waterbirth – although the picture is not complete'. Breathing is inhibited through natural physiological processes, including hormones (prostaglandins, progesterone and endorphins) released from the placenta and a low metabolic rate. This process is further supported by the large number of chemoreceptors found in the larynx of the newborn, which is said to facilitate the baby into recognizing which fluids can be swallowed and which inhaled. In other words, the baby recognises that it should not inhale water but that it can be swallowed. This reflex is seen by many practitioners who undertake waterbirths and have not seen inhalation of water. The one cautionary tale is in the case of severe intrapartum hypoxia, not the normal physiological hypoxia of labour but severe, where the fetus may be compromised and this mechanism can be overridden.

Table 8.1: Stimuli mimics for delaying respiration

TRIGGER IN AIR	WATERBIRTH MIMIC
Environment	
Room temperature 21°C-22°C	Water temperature 37-37.5°C
Gravity	
Full force in air	Gravitation less in water
Tactile	
Delivery technique Suctioning	Non-touch technique No suctioning
Auditory	
Sounds of people and delivery	Muffled sounds at delivery
Chemoreceptors	
Stimulated with hypoxia. Triggered with clamping/ cutting of cord	No stimuli in water, if term, healthy baby. Cord not cut until immersion. Sited in larynx and sensitive to type of fluid
Closure of temporary structures	
Triggered following clamping/cutting of cord. Changes in chemical and mechanics of circulation	No stimuli until cord clamped and cut, and first breath taken
Pressure sensors	
Triggered by delivery technique and gravity	Non-touch technique. Gravitational- less environment
Heads reflex	
Triggered by first lung expansion	Not triggered until lungs expand in air

Fetal adaptation to extrauterine life

It has been suggested by many authors that it is a multifactorial stimulus that is responsible for triggering respiration. These stimuli, shown in Table 8.1 (cited Burke, 1985; Hamed *et al*, 1967), can be mimicked for a moment in time to slightly delay the initiation of respiration.

If these protective reflexes are altered in any way, i.e. a need to assist with the delivery due to shoulder dystocia, initiation of respiration may be triggered and the planned waterbirth reassessed. Similarly, if fetal compromise occurs during labour then the resultant changes may preclude a water labour/birth (see Chapter Ten).

Studies have been undertaken on lambs to assist in identifying the stimuli to respiration and other physiological issues surrounding water labour/birth. It must be assumed that one reason for the use of sheep is the ethical and practical issues that arise from these studies (Falconer and Powless, 1982; Hamed *et al*, 1967).

Evidence from Johnson (1996) supports clinical practice regarding the safe use of waterbirth for low risk mothers/babies. Johnson's work centres around why babies do not breathe underwater, the main themes being:

- hormonal – influenced by prostaglandin E2

- warm fetal environment

- fetal metabolism – minimal active thermogenesis or heat production in utero

- fetal hypoxia – inhibits fetal breathing, unless severe when gasping occurs

- fetal in utero environment – 'recognition' of its own and foreign fluids

- fetal larynx response – reduced diving response of bradycardia and hypertension.

This notion of newborn's not breathing underwater is further supported by Eldering *et al* (cited Beech 1996).

So if water has the properties described in this chapter, does it mean that the baby develops differently postnatally? Unsubstantiated work quoted by Ray (1986) states:

that with water training programmes these children... are more confident, lack aggression, are more intelligent, rarely fall sick and easily withstand cold and weather changes.

She continues:

that they are said to have no temper tantrums, sleep soundly, are physically stronger, more active, brighter and resourceful.

These type of claims, when not substantiated and clearly studied, do little for the waterbirth movement.

Apgar scoring

Recent articles have again raised questions regarding fetal monitoring and perhaps more interestingly Apgar scores. Debating the use of this score in Crozier and Sinclair (1999) brings to the forefront the many variables that can affect the actual score given (gestational age, maternal analgesia and subjective scoring by the person assigning the score).

The paper continues with the question that there is poor correlation between Apgar score and umbilical blood pH. Suggestions that the one-minute Apgar score is often measured earlier than one full minute, is supported both by clinical experience and teaching undertaken by myself.

I suggest that midwives watch a 'normal' dry birth, prior to waterbirths, and observe the normal physiological adaptation to ex-utero life. In other words, actually time one full minute and then assign an Apgar score. This simple exercise is often a revelation to us as midwives, since often I find the one-minute score is assigned either at birth, or at less than one minute.

Following this exercise, observation of waterbirths (both clinically and on video) highlight the apparent time it takes for a baby to cry and respond. A minute is a very long time in a newborn's life!

Comparison of Apgar scores are often quoted in publications (Beech 1996) and in audit papers (Garland and Jones 1994 and 1997). Does this really reflect what actually occurs at birth?

Conclusion

The fetal viewpoint and perspective is indeed worth further investigation. How do we proceed and offer the research or studies that will provide the evidence to future generations? Morris (1991, p.117) seems to sum up my own view of this issue by writing:

> *Despite its advantages to both mother and baby, many doctors dislike this type of labour because it is more difficult for them to take charge of the events that occur inside the pool. If the birth is a normal healthy one, their objections are groundless but if complications are likely that is another matter. With modern technology (and skilled care givers – my wording) however, it should not be too difficult to predict what kind of delivery to expect and to act accordingly.*

CHAPTER NINE

Research issues for midwives using water in practice

Changing Childbirth (Department of Health, 1993) stated:

> *There is a long history in maternity services of well-intentioned changes which are not backed up with proper research-based evidence to support their introduction... this is also true for other techniques and practices such as waterbirth, homeopathy and aromatherapy... where women express a wish for a particular form of care which has no proven benefit, this fact must be discussed with them openly and fairly. (p.63, 4.3.1)*

I agree with this viewpoint and feel that as only an estimated ten per cent of obstetrical procedures in use are researched satisfactorily (WHO), it is imperative that those of us who introduce new procedures ensure that adequate evaluation takes place. Procedures such as ultrasound, routine fetal monitoring and epidurals have all hit the press in varying degrees over the past few years with reports that are contradictory.

When I first started waterbirth, it soon became apparent that little documented evidence existed as to the advantages or disadvantages of using water. I relied on colleagues to keep hand held, and then computerised records, to start the evaluation and audit programme. A true randomised controlled trial has on many occasions been suggested but I have an ethical dilemma with this concept and concerns about this type of trial have been published (Baum, 1993). It is also apparent that clinical trials would require funding and consumer input, a fact identified recently through an AIMS article (Robinson, 1994).

Over the years midwives who have undertaken water labours/births have kept clear records of the care in labour and delivery. Objective data measuring length of labour, perineal trauma, Apgar scores and blood loss have been reported by several authors (Burns and Greenish, 1993; Garland and Jones, 1994) who published data from two units in Oxford and Maidstone. How can we expect to challenge medical interventions and routine procedures, if we are not willing to audit any new midwifery practices? In 1986, Flint wrote about the way, as practitioners, we could challenge routine hospital procedures. When we introduced waterbirths at Maidstone we included all professionals thought to have a view on this topic. The 'challenging' aspect was never an issue since everyone felt included and participatory in service development. See Chapter Eleven for details of various accounts written by those involved in service provision.

Accountability and research appear to me to be inherently linked. As practitioners we must ensure that our practice is research-based and up-to-date. To be accountable for our actions we are charged with the task of having knowledge that allows us to weigh up the relative benefits of different treatments. We constantly make clinical judgements that decide with our clients whether a particular therapy is required for her care. Some decisions have far-reaching consequences, for example HIV testing and amniocentesis, whilst others are based on current evaluation of the situation, such as should this woman have an artificial rupture of membranes (ARM). So, in order for us to remain research-based we need two things, up-to-date information and continuing education. Formats for both already exist in midwifery. Statutory refresher courses are now more flexible and geared to individual needs. We are also fortunate in having access to several databases including MIDIRS and RCM.

Another reason for auditing and evaluating our practice is to formulate the type of research that we wish to follow. It became very evident early in Maidstone's experience that the length of labour starting from the point that the mother requested pain relief was shorter in the waterbirth group. I thus started the first part of our research with this in mind. Before I highlight what objective and subjective data could be measured it is worth reviewing what others have said about research in the light of new innovations in childbirth. McCraw (1989) writes:

Throughout the struggles over [these] innovations in childbirth, proponents have all too often made broad, sweeping and unsupported claims about the lasting benefits of these changes;

similarly, opponents have frequently predicted dire calamities, also with limited supporting evidence, if such innovations are adopted. Advocates of the status quo have both the power of tradition and the weight of inertia on their side; it thus behoves proponents of changes to demonstrate that their innovations are both safe and beneficial. It is naive to assume that mere anecdotal evidence or assertions that their innovation is 'more natural' will lead to its adoption by a medical profession that prides itself on its objectivity and scientific method.

This attitude to research appears to me to be the way forward. As I have already stated, too many other interventions have been introduced without adequate research. To introduce another procedure without fulfilling this remit would seem foolhardy and not without its own share of criticism. I wrote in Chapter Four about professional visits to other units in America and Europe and shared with you the type of questions that I ask when with these practitioners.

Suggested questions to ask of other units

- What sort of parent education and/or preparation of parents occurs prior to offering water labour/birth?
- Is there a cost implication for clients, i.e. are they asked to hire a tub or buy a liner for the tub?
- What education/training/ground rules are set up for staff?
- What sort of tubs are available to the women? Is a list available for local tub hire?
- Is an agreed criteria for use available to clients and staff?
- What is the ratio of Primip:Multip use?
- Is the woman permitted to add anything to the water, i.e. aromatherapy oils, and if yes, who administers this?
- What water temperature is recommended?
- How are mother and baby monitored?
- How is the third stage managed, i.e. physiological or active?
- What outcomes are being audited by the unit and how?

Research undertaken by other authors

Over the past few years many units and individuals have started to publish data that promotes evidence-based practice. However, many of these studies lack validity because of the generalisation of their findings. Comparison between data was difficult because of the differences in the methods of data collection and analysis.

The major exponents of waterbirth have written about the subject in a variety of journals, although some have been reviewed by others, due to language problems. Texts that are worth reviewing include Balaskas and Gordon (1990), Lichy and Herzburg (1993), Odent (1983, 1990), Johnson and Odent (1994), Harper (1994), Tjarkovsky (cited in Sidenbladh, 1983).

It is generally agreed that there is very little 'hard' evidence as to the advantages or disadvantages of water labour/birth. There are some notable articles, which should be reviewed by professionals wishing to undertake waterbirths. Eriksson *et al* 1996, Garland and Jones 1997, Aird *et al* 1997 and Brown 1998 all warrant some reading, in light of the current evidence being accumulated. Whilst there is a growing number of reports of personal experiences, from both midwives and mothers, they have little scientific value. The subjective use of these reports should not, however, be undervalued and in themselves can provide immense information for use as professionals (see Chapter Eleven).

Notable studies and research articles

The use of randomised controlled trials is often argued as a suitable methodology for studying waterbirths. However, an article by Bothamley and Chadwick (cited Beech 1996), discusses the potential problems encountered when planning research into issues surrounding waterbirths. They rightly assert that research could be fraught with difficulties on both ethical and pragmatic matters. Any research should first safeguard individual rights and second, facilitate research that is aimed at improving treatment and care (Lilford, cited Beech 1996). It is clear that the difficulties surrounding waterbirth research would need to overcome the problems of unit/midwife/client self-selection, women's desire for choice and finding enough participants who would be willing to enter into a randomised controlled trial.

Rush *et al*, 1996

This study, undertaken in Canada, investigated 392 labours of women offered a tub (whirlpool) for labour, to review clinical outcomes. This randomised controlled trial investigated both water and dry labour, but waterbirth was not offered. The authors concluded that whirlpool baths in labour had a positive effect on analgesia requirements, instrumental rates, condition of perineum and personal satisfaction. Interestingly, especially as a whirlpool bath was used, there were no significant differences between maternal and newborn infections, or between dry and water labours. Despite these findings, most waterbirth practitioners do not advocate the use of jacuzzis because of the problem of cleaning when potentially used by many women.

Hall and Holloway, 1998

Although only a small piece of grounded theory approached research (9 women), the work further supports many stories published about women's experiences of using water for labour or delivery. Examples are, Parkes and Fernandes, UK 1998 and Schreuder, USA 1996.

All of the women except one stated that water was beneficial and that they felt more in control. They valued their own involvement in determining the outcome of their care (see Chapter Twelve). It reports that water was a positive experience for this group of healthy women.

Two studies that look at the issue of infection are Hawkins (1995) and Anderson (1996). In Hawkins, 32 women were studied – 16 in water and 16 non-water. They had pre- and post-delivery screening. The results showed more micro organisms (15 compared to 10 dry births) in the waterbirth group. However, interestingly, none of the babies showed clinical signs of infection, and were colonised with *Staphylococcus aureus* and one case of *E. Coli*. Whilst the author comments on the need for infection audit and cleaning policies, one wonders how many other births in a normal maternity unit would yield colonisation of bacterium?

In Anderson *et al*, a larger study, 317 water labours and 312 dry labours were compared. There is a reported increase in maternal infections. However, actual figures are not published, but there were no differences in neonatal infections. All infections were treated and there were no long term sequlea. As the actual numbers are not reproduced it is impossible to relate these findings to clinical practice, and thus the value of the work is somewhat lost.

Infection control and birthing pools

- Consider at risk groups in own locality and thus screening procedures.
- Involve infection control and the microbiology department early in the planning stages.

- Ensure universal precautions are used with all women using the pool.
- The pool should be cleaned daily (plumbed in) whether used or not. Home pools should always follow the manufacturer's instructions for cleaning, and use of disposable liners.
- Pools should be cleaned and dried after each individual use.
- All equipment should be sterilised, disposable, or able to be cheaply replaced.
- Audit forms should be completed with a monitoring system in situ when an infection occurs, to review policies.
- Positive feedback should be given to all practitioners on the use of the pool.

In 1999 at the ICM (International Confederation of Midwives) conference in Manila, several papers of interest were presented. Lisbeth Nyman from Denmark highlighted the risk of infection following waterbirths. This study of 200 women (100 water and 100 dry births) showed no increased infection rates between the two groups. All mothers and babies were deemed low risk, uncomplicated pregnancies, at term, singleton, cephalic presentation and ruptured membranes less than 24 hours.

Another interesting paper by Elizabeth Cluett from the University of Southampton discussed the findings, and potential for future studies, of using water in first stage dystocia. This small study (17 women) concluded by stating:

> ... labouring in water was more effective at facilitating labour than conservative management (i.e. do nothing) and only slightly less effective than augmentation.

I await the full trial with great interest, especially in today's consumer-led service, where many women are seeking the lowest possible intervention rates. Would they view the use of water for first stage dystocia as intervention?

A national study of labour and birth in water

The National Perinatal Epidemiology Unit (NPEU) was commissioned in August 1993 by the Department of Health to undertake an urgent survey of current practice in waterbirths. This followed a review by McCandlish and Renfrew (1993).

The aims of the survey are:

- To assess current practices and use of birthing pools in England and Wales.
- To provide estimates of the number of women who have used immersion in water during labour and/or birth.
- To assess problems encountered using immersion in water.
- To collect information on policies for pool use, resource implications and any evaluations that have taken place.
- To assess the feasibility of carrying out more formal evaluation such as a randomised controlled trial.

The study was in two parts, with an initial questionnaire sent out to all heads of midwifery in England and Wales. This established an overview of current practice in provider units. A telephone interview was then conducted, to collect information on the number of women using water, details of current practice, problems encountered and costs involved in service provision.

Proposed outcome measures
- Pain and need for pain relief
- Length of labour
- Mode of delivery
- Perineal trauma
- Post-partum haemorrhage
- Admission to SCBU
- Infection of mother, baby or care giver
- Resource use

1995 update
Following an initial questionnaire, which was sent to all provider units in England and Wales during December 1993, the second stage of the survey was a telephone interview. The NPEU looked at current usage and practice, collected guidelines where these were available and the financial implications for use of water.

In April 1995 the NPEU reported in the *BJM* the results of the study. It is not within my remit to fully describe the results but the authors (Alderdice *et al*, 1995) concluded by stating:

There is no evidence from this survey to suggest that labour and birth in water should not continue to be offered as an option to women in England and Wales. Questions remain, however, about the possible benefits and hazards, the conditions of practice and resource use. A randomised controlled trial could address some of these issues.

British Paediatric Surveillance Unit (BPSU)

This study was started in April 1994 and ran until April 1995. The study has been set up in response to reports of perinatal death or damage following, although not necessarily caused by, labour or delivery in water. The study aimed to:

- Estimate the incidence of adverse neonatal outcome in babies delivered in water.

- Identify babies who are admitted to special care or die, following labour in water, to examine whether there is evidence that the use of water during labour is associated with adverse outcome.

The study is further broken down on the reporting format as:

- Any perinatal death:
  - following delivery in water

  - following labour in water.

- Any admission to special care unit within 48 hours of birth:
  - following delivery in water
  - following labour in water.

This survey has been reported in *BJM*, August 1999, by Gilbert and Tookey. They conclude that after some 4032 waterbirths in England and Wales (0.6 per cent of all deliveries):

Our study provides good evidence that, for women who deliver in water, perinatal mortality is not substantially increased compared with low risk women delivering on dry land. The data are compatible with a small increase (relative risk less than 3.6) or decrease in perinatal mortality for deliveries in water compared with those on dry land.

Local research at Maidstone

To facilitate credibility within my profession, I decided that it was important to undertake some research within the unit that I worked. The study was retrospective and involved only women who fulfilled the unit's normality criteria. The information was collected through the unit's delivery register and not from client held records. Three groups were studied:

- Non immersion group (those women who chose another form of pain relief)

- First stage immersion group (those women who entered the water but left during labour)

- Waterbirth group (women who chose to remain in the water).

Since the study was retrospective, women were not assigned randomly to the groups.

Outcomes considered

- *Duration of labour.* In the study we compared three groups of women as stated above. The starting point of labour was taken from the point where the woman requested pain relief. The vaginal examination nearest to this point was taken as the onset of active labour and thus the measurement of length of first and second stage combined. It was important to use this starting point, since it was the only marker that could be shown to be the same in all women. The point at which she chooses her preferred method of analgesia was either water or not. The clients all fell within the same criteria, i.e. at term, singleton and cephalic presentation. No known or envisaged complications were expected. Exclusions to this criteria were those women who required syntocinon, since they would not be allowed to use the water for pain relief. Due to the timespan of the work, the ages and social classes of the women were similar as were the clinical practices within the unit. The only discrepancy was the change of staff over the seven year period. I do not feel that this factor played any significant role, since the senior staff (grades H and I) have not altered.

- *Use of drugs during labour and delivery.* As part of the study we reviewed what forms of pain relief were utilised by the women who did not choose water. For those women who started with the tub but then left and opted for another mode of analgesia (either by choice or necessity – see reasons for leaving water) the outcome of pain relief was recorded. The relative benefits of water over any other form of pain relief has already been described in Chapter Seven. Suffice to state here that all forms of pain relief have cost resources for the unit and potential implications for maternal and newborn physiology.

- *Perineal trauma rates.* Episiotomy was not performed on the waterbirth clients. Because of this the rate of perineal tears tended to be higher. There is, of course, much debate regarding whether tears or episiotomy suture and heal better. I do not feel that this book should address these issues but it is certainly worth reviewing the literature. The study that was published highlighted an increased intact perineum rate in the waterbirth clients. This was not reported by other authors (Burns and Greenish, 1993) but this may in part be due to interpretation of their data (no distinction was made between the waterbirth and first stage immersion group).

- *Post-partum haemorrhage rates.* In this study the groups were not quite compatible. The waterbirth group were offered a physiological third stage, whilst the dry land and water immersion groups had an active third stage. It is important to bear this in mind when reviewing the data but allowing for this difference, the study's main objective to show non compromise in mother appears to be borne out. The waterbirth group had slightly higher rates of post-partum haemorrhage (allowing for what has been said in Chapter Ten about blood loss). The biggest issue I feel is that the midwife undertaking physiological third stage is confident performing this procedure.

- *Incidence of low Apgar scores.* The baseline for measuring low Apgar scores was a marker of < 6/1 minute. This criteria was felt to be an indicator of fetal compromise. In the study we found that there were significantly fewer low Apgars in the primip and multip groups, as compared with the other two groups. Again the original issue was to show that we were not compromising newborns by offering waterbirth.

This study needs duplicating in both my own unit and in other units in order to show if indeed these results are to be considered valid (Garland and Jones, 1994).

Waterbirth labour audit form versus dry birth

1st stage	2nd stage	perineum	apgar	EBL	analgesia	TOS	Delivery type	Para	Cervix	Age group	Age	Ethnic group	Left water reason

Codes required for:
Analgesia / Delivery type / Age group / Ethnic group / Left water

Potential areas for research

Over the last seven years I have been gathering ideas for potential areas of research. Many could easily be undertaken by any midwife or unit doing waterbirths, others would require resources such as computer space and researcher input to analyse data. Bearing this in mind does not, however, stop us from utilizing our clinical experiences in the form of audit and evaluation.

Potential areas for research include the following:

- Aquanatal preparation – does this make any difference to uptake or use of water labour/birth?

- Uterine activity – during immersion versus: water temperature; length of immersion; total length of labour?

- Pain relief – what quality and quantity of pain relief is measurable in these client groups?

- Delivery outcomes – Mode of delivery
  - Perineal trauma
  - Apgar scores
  - Blood loss
  - Third stage management

- Primip versus Multip uptake

- Cost effectiveness

- Breastfeeding rates – do more women start and long term breastfeed?

- Infection rates – maternal and newborn

- Management of complications

- Adverse outcomes

- SCBU admission rates

- Subjective comments from parents

- Midwife comments and experiences

- Uptake patterns – why does one get three deliveries in one day and then no one using the tub for a week?

- Postnatal depression rates

- Length of postnatal hospital stay

This type of local work is invaluable since it assists midwives in auditing their own individual practices. However, since 1998 a collaborative study has been supported through the NHS executive research and development fund, to expand local work to a national country-wide study. At this point in time, the first year's work is being produced and will be published in midwifery texts and at conference presentations.

Conclusion

This research chapter has been aimed at highlighting the need to continue the audit and evaluation side of water labour/birth. For those midwives interested in research there are a wealth of opportunities to expand the parameters of clinical care. McCraw (1989) sums up the issue of waterbirth research by writing:

> If waterbirth or any other innovation in childbirth proves anxiety reducing or otherwise more pleasurable for the couple and not dangerous to the fetus, that is enough and it should be available as an option. It is not necessary that it results in a new breed of human. Such scientifically unsupported claims leave one open to questions of honesty and ethics, if not litigation, in today's society. What should always be kept in mind, it seems to this writer, is informed freedom of choice. Replacing an inflexible system that does not allow waterbirth with one that would require every woman to labour and deliver in a tub of water is surely no improvement.

CHAPTER TEN

What if...?

As a practising midwife one of the greatest concerns is the possibility of complications or emergencies occurring in the water. This chapter has been enlarged to cover new clinical situations and the professional issues that have occurred since waterbirths first became popular in the UK. Here I share with you the practical issues surrounding complications or problems that may occur in water labour or birth. When I first started undertaking waterbirth it was by reviewing my Code of Practice and discussion with Jasmine Callow, Director of Midwifery from 1986–1989, that I came to several conclusions about where I stood.

With any potential complication we all know as midwives that early detection or avoidance is the best plan. But it is also true that even in the most normal pregnancy, labour and delivery, unforeseen problems do occur. Water is not the panacea for all evils, and midwives and parents need to be aware that whatever can occur on dry land can occur in the water. I believe that four main issues should be reviewed with regard to complications prior to starting a waterbirth service.

- Are there physiological areas that need to be highlighted, for example, can you clamp and cut the cord under water?
- Are the mechanisms of labour altered by the complication?
- Will your colleagues support you if unforeseen complications occur?
- Would you have time to empty the water? It is often quicker to ask the mother to stand up. Lagoon tubs take 10–15 minutes to empty.

These issues are vital as they may cause us to rethink how we deal with problems and we may actually need to relearn or adapt our clinical skills.

As stated in Chapter Five, peer support played a huge role in starting the waterbirths at Maidstone. When problems do occur – and by the law of averages they will – it is really important that we feel supported by both colleagues and parents. The following case highlights this situation well.

Clinical scenario – peer and parental support

Janet had a waterbirth in 1990 under my care and returned two years later for another water labour and birth. Labour started spontaneously and had progressed normally. She entered the water at 4cm dilated, with full dilation apparent two and a half hours later.

Maternal and fetal observations were within normal limits with clear liquor draining. The baby's head delivered without intervention, and I waited for restitution (external rotation of the head, internal rotation of shoulders). After several moments and after one large contraction, the shoulders failed to deliver. I therefore slipped my finger down and felt a tight cord around the baby's neck. It was not loose enough to loop over the head or deliver the baby through, so I asked Janet to stand up and allow me to deliver the shoulders after clamping and cutting the cord on 'terra firma'!

Baby Jonathan was delivered safely with the next contraction after I had clamped and cut the cord, which was actually wrapped around him three times. Apgar scores were 8/1 and 10/5. He was wrapped up and given to Janet who then proceeded to deliver the placenta spontaneously.

One hour after delivery he started to 'grunt' and the paediatrician was asked to see him as he was showing some signs of nasal flaring. The doctor decided to admit Jonathan to the Special Care Baby Unit (SCBU), where he had a full infection screen. The diagnosis recorded in the notes was 'Fetal distress caused by waterbirth'. Naturally I was extremely concerned about the diagnosis since the baby was not actually delivered in water.

The moral of the story is this. The consultant happened to be on SCBU at the time I saw the diagnosis, and after having seen the baby and speaking to both myself as the midwife at delivery and the admitting doctor, he altered the diagnosis. There were no repercussions for baby or midwife and the support from the consultant made this a good learning experience rather than a negative one.

Maternal choice vs political/professional conflict

During the last couple of years there have been instances of a conflict arising between women and professionals when the woman's preferred choice of delivery was not the political/professional one on offer. This was shown graphically by the media in the case of the East Herts Midwives (Editorial 1994). Whilst it is outside the scope of this book to comment on this intricate incident, it does highlight the potential problems that may exist when a mother requests a waterbirth in an area in which there may be a conflict between her and the Trust. The two midwives in this case appear to have been caught somewhere in the middle.

So what if... you have a mother requesting a waterbirth when your unit is unable to provide this type of care? Whilst both the UKCC (1995) and the RCM (1994) clearly regard waterbirths as part of normal, albeit, adapted midwifery practice, this is not always the case in practice. As midwives, we have a professional responsibility to provide care for this woman; we also have a responsibility to ensure that we have the appropriate skills and education to undertake this role.

As discussed in Chapters One and Eleven, professional and educational services are provided. I believe this is the responsibility of both individuals and/or the Trusts for which we work. This service should provide both educational opportunities and the development/adapting of clinical skills. A simple flow chart may assist midwives in supporting mothers through this choice. (See Figure 10.1.)

If this type of negotiation occurs, then by taking a partnership approach to planning care I have found most mothers are able to receive the type of care they wish. This unfortunately is not always the case. Robinson (1996) writes that a woman may be attracted to a particular unit because it has a pool, but when she actually wishes to use the pool finds that it is 'not available'. In other words, a carrot on a stick scenario. A similar article, again by Robinson, published in the *British Journal of Midwifery* (1996), discussed the politics of pool use. Robinson concludes:

> *We know that birth will never be risk free, but we want reliable evidence of risks and benefits, and then judge them and choose according to our own priorities.*

This reinforces the need for audit, education, written evidence and development of clinical skills, all of which midwives are producing.

Cord snapping

Whilst, of course, potentially very serious, this issue has only occurred on two occasions in my clinical practice. In both situations there was no way the midwives could have foreseen any problem. There was no fetal distress and no delay in shoulder rotation or delivery.

In my experience, neither babies were compromised, since the midwife was able to 'catch' and then clamp the cord before a major blood leakage. Neither cord appeared particularly short, and one might therefore assume that wherever the mother had delivered the cord could have 'snapped'.

Fetal hyperthermia

Controversy still surrounds the problems that were encountered with two babies in Bristol in 1993 after the mothers had laboured in water. The issue raised following this scenario was regarding in utero fetal hyperthermia. The previous edition of this book highlighted the importance of ensuring that maternal and thus fetal hyperthermia does not occur. (See Appendix II.)

A paper by Charles (1998) explores the physiological adaptation that occurs if the mother becomes overheated. In my experience, the risk of hyperthermia can be greatly reduced by giving good clear guidelines for an ambient room, recording maternal and water temperatures, and by encouraging maternal hydration and a regular change of position (particularly to facilitate upper torso out of water).

I have only been aware of one mother becoming pyrexial. On being unable to lower her temperature she was asked to leave the water; the baby delivered quickly after this with no obvious compromise.

Neonatal polycythaemia

An article by Austin *et al* (1997) is of interest since it appears to be the only incident dealing with polycythaemia in a newborn. The article has implications for the way we manage physiological third stage and what information is given to parents. In physiological third stage there is a delay in clamping of the cord following delivery. This is associated with high PCV and plasma viscosity. However, as the authors rightly state, there have been no other reports of polycythaemia.

The umbilical cord should vasoconstrict on contact with air, but if the cord remains in warm water for a prolonged period the physiology may alter, causing polycythaemia. In my twelve years of experience I and several other well established practitioners, have never experienced this phenomena. Whilst this situation could occur, clinical skills and experience do not appear to bear out this potential problem.

As midwives we certainly should be aware of and evaluate all potential issues. In the light of this one client, I do not know of any established practitioners who have altered their practice.

Fig 10.1: Supporting women through choice

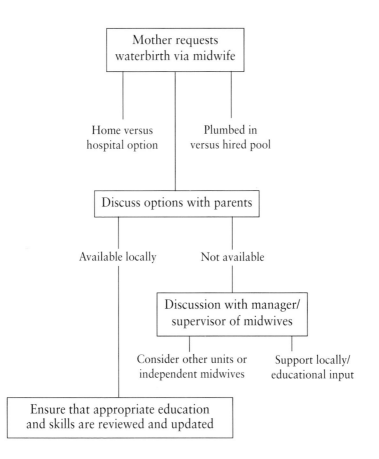

Poor publicity: 'Death of the water babies'

During 1993 several reports appeared in the media regarding the death of a water baby in Sweden. This incident, which made the front pages of every national newspaper in England, highlighted the problems that midwives can experience with negative publicity. Many units who were about to, or had just started a waterbirthing service, stopped offering it overnight and in some units even stopped offering water labour.

This caused a great many problems, not least of all for those women who had booked this option for their delivery. It was an increasingly difficult time for those of us who continued with waterbirths, as we struggled to keep abreast of the little professional information we had about this very tragic case.

Many units did continue with their service, and this was one of many times where the unique 'networking' that has developed with waterbirth practitioners found its true outlet.

Negative publicity is never easy to deal with, but we should always balance our own practice and audits, with the national and international viewpoints. As practitioners, we need to realise that negative stories make news and all the positive accounts do not, so read the media, but accept that good news is not newsworthy to the popular press.

Labour/birth in water is not just a mode of pain relief or delivery, but an attitude to care. This type of attitude supports the way that we wish to work as professionals, as partners in care, with opportunities to learn from and with each other. In my experience women leave the water for three main reasons:

- failure of analgesia
- fetal distress, or
- failure to progress.

It has always been my policy to ensure that a discussion of all the advantages and disadvantages of water labour/birth takes place, as part of the couple's pre-education, including why women leave the tubs.

Having established a base, all other observations follow normal midwifery care and deviation from normal is referred to a medical practitioner, as stated in the *Midwives Code of Practice* 1998 (UKCC, 1998).

Reasons for leaving water or possible complications

Fetal distress

Gibb and Arulkumaran (1992, p.67) discuss the value of a 20-minute base admission trace. In a low-risk woman it was reported that following a normal cardiotocograph (CTG) intermittent auscultation with a further trace 2-3 hours later was an acceptable standard for practice. Interpretation is vital and as midwives we should ensure that we are confident in our CTG skills.

Having this standard enables us to offer water labour and birth to low-risk women in our care. Intermittent auscultation is possible with the newest line in monitoring (see Useful Addresses). It appears that the most helpful are dopplers that actually go under water, thereby reducing disturbance to the labouring women.

If any sign of fetal compromise becomes apparent the woman is asked to leave the water or stand up if delivery is imminent (trying to climb out at this stage is not only difficult but could be dangerous).

Meconium-stained liquor

Despite the debate regarding meconium-stained liquor, it appears that most professionals feel that this is potentially a sign of fetal compromise. It is estimated that meconium is present in 15 per cent of all deliveries and up to 40 per cent in post-mature labours. Meconium aspiration may cause in utero fetal heart changes and possible dangers to the baby at delivery, necessitating continuous monitoring during labour and intervention at delivery with rapid sucking (often on the perineum). The risk assessment status of this has now altered and women should not stay in the water in these circumstances (Gibb, 1988; Cronk and Flint, 1989).

Water contamination

This issue causes some alarm amongst colleagues, both from the aesthetic and practical viewpoint. It is not pleasant for mother or midwife if the water is contaminated with faeces or blood, and the water should be cleared with a sieve or fish net (see 'Equipment' in Chapter Five).

If the water is very 'murky' then it is probably best to ask the woman to leave the water, clean out the tub and start again. Practically, it is difficult to estimate blood loss if the water is already murky, and one described factor in the death of the Swedish baby was faecal contamination.

Robinson (1994) and Rosser (1994) both reported on this issue. The physiological basis for this is not clear, but it may be due to a change in the bacterial flora at delivery. Although the baby is usually colonised with his mother's own bacterial flora, the alien nature of faeces may alter this fine interplay between mother and baby.

In early waterbirths in America some tubs had sea salt added to them in an attempt to make it more saline and possibly closer to amniotic fluid and provide a bacteriostatic solution. This practice does not appear relevant or necessary (Harper, 1994, p.160).

Failure to progress

As already stated, water is not the panacea for all evils, and just as labours can be slower or stop out of water so is true in water. I do not advocate that all normal labouring women require the use of a cervical dilation curve on the partogram, but as midwives we are well aware of the physical and psychological stresses placed on women during labour. Changes to the woman's body are normal in labour and each of us will tolerate different lengths of first and second stage. Just as we will all deal with different amounts of fatigue and stress, so each woman is individual and should be treated as such in labour. The point of this with water labour and waterbirth is that as each woman is an individual, so her labour should be cared for, within the normal parameters set by ourselves as autonomous practitioners, or within the maternity units where we work. Fundamental changes to normal practice may need to be made in units where active management of labour prevails (Crawford, 1987).

If labour is not 'progressing' the woman may need to leave the water and mobilise, possibly eat and drink, and facilitate increased contractions. Complementary therapies may assist this process (Tiran and Mack, 1994).

Maternal hyperthermia

For the mother to maintain her core temperature it is vital that she is able to lose heat through four main avenues: conduction, convection, evaporation and radiation (see Appendix II). The mother should be encouraged to drink large amounts of fluid and her temperature should be recorded regularly. An ambient temperature within the room will also assist in maintaining a normal core temperature. If the mother becomes hyperthermic and tachycardic her baby will also react to this change in internal environment. This interdependency is further shown in Appendix I.

Often when women become too hot in the birthing tubs they have not been encouraged to drink, the room is very hot and they are sitting deep in the tub, i.e. their upper torso is not out of the water.

Nuchal cord

One of the most difficult situations we are faced with as midwives is when the cord is wrapped around the baby's neck. The basic principle states that if the cord has caused no fetal compromise during labour, which you would be aware of from auscultation of the fetal heart rate, then it is unlikely to cause problems at delivery.

Some colleagues do not feel for the cord at delivery because of this basic assumption. I only feel for the cord if the baby fails to deliver with the next contraction. If it is around the neck I either slip it over the head or deliver the baby through the loop – this was a new skill that I had to learn. As a student I was taught that if the cord could not be looped over, then it was clamped and cut. This is not an option with waterbirth since it could trigger respiration or stimulate the baby by tactile stimulation (see Chapter Eight).

It is also worthwhile considering delivering the baby with the membranes intact; although a rare occurrence, in my experience this is a difficult situation to handle. I have found that if the membranes are still intact as the head is about to be delivered, they should be ruptured at this time. If the baby delivers in the cawl (although considered to be lucky) it is very difficult to break once in air. Not only is it difficult, but very fiddly and slippery and could cause more problems than it is worth.

Shoulder dystocia

When I speak to colleagues this is often the first concern expressed. Just how do you deal with this situation in water? The same principles exist in water as on dry land – rotate and tilt the mother's pelvis to facilitate the rotation of the baby's shoulders (Cronk and Flint, 1989, p.159). The first difference in water is the physiological stimulation to the baby and the potential of tactile stimuli under water triggering respiration. Second, is the practical issue of moving mother in water. It is often thought to be easier as water encourages mobility, it may be that one moves the mother in water, or that she stands and delivers in a supported/leaning position.

This is one time when it is good to have practised the practicalities prior to the event. Parent education also pays dividends at this time. I have never had to ask a mother twice to stand up, usually she has done it before I have finished my request.

Episiotomy

The Midwives Code of Practice (1991, p.3, 2.2.6) states that as midwives we should be able to perform episiotomies when required. It is this interpretation that often causes dilemmas when caring for women. Some midwives and maternity units may have an active attitude to performing this procedure. Good evidence exists to show that episiotomies are not always the answer and that much debate will continue about which sutures or heals better. The long-term consequences of episiotomy should not be overlooked from the mother's point of view. I believe that there are times when an episiotomy is required. In an emergency an episiotomy may well facilitate delivery but if that is occurring, I would question why the mother is still in the water. I do not, therefore, advocate that episiotomy is performed underwater.

Post-partum haemorrhage

This situation is difficult to deal with and runs parallel with estimating blood loss at a waterbirth. How do you measure blood loss in 180 gallons of water? The scientific way is to use an optical density probe, but these cost around £700, and knowing how often ordinary thermometers are broken I can imagine the situation being similar with this piece of equipment.

Initially I tried hard to think how we could estimate blood loss and I soon came to the conclusion that the actual amount was not the important issue. The important thing is the way that the mother copes with her blood loss, not the amount that she has lost.

We all know that if five midwives are asked to estimate the same amount of loss we end up with five different answers. Estimating loss has sometimes been called 'guestimating' because of this. Each mother will tolerate a different amount of 'normal' blood loss which will depend on many factors: her own antenatal haemoglobin; her body reserves; length of labour; and probably genetic makeup. Gyte (1992) produced an interesting paper on this subject.

How many times have you visited a mother on the postnatal ward who has lost 650ml and found her fit and well, breastfeeding and helping with the tea trolley, and then visited a mother who apparently lost 450ml the day before, and she feels and looks awful and has no energy to breastfeed her baby. I am certain you can all recall similar stories. This is the mother's ability to cope with a normal amount of blood loss at delivery. This attitude prevails at waterbirths, I do not record the estimated blood loss in any other terms than <500ml unless the mother is compromised, i.e. pallor, clammy, thready pulse, low blood pressure or reports other physical signs. In other words this woman is not having a post-partum haemorrhage. This way of recording blood loss may need negotiation in maternity units or with supervisors who are used to seeing a definitive figure. It now acts as part of the RCM's position paper (RCM, 1994).

Post-partum haemorrhage is dealt with outside the water with an oxytocic drug as appropriate. It is worth remembering that with the vasodilatation that occurs in water, third stage management in water may appear to lead to an increased blood loss.

I have never experienced any difficulty in getting a mother out of the tub. The few excessive blood losses recorded have often been when physiological third-stage management has been hastened. I have never seen a collapsed mother, in or out of the tub at any waterbirth I have attended. A lifting sling is available from Silverlea Textiles (see Useful Addresses).

Suturing

As a student I was always taught to repair a tear or episiotomy as soon as possible after delivery, but it became apparent that this was not appropriate following waterbirth. The perineal tissue appears to become 'waterlogged' and it is important to allow time to revitalise the skin and muscle layers. If you try to suture too soon after delivery you may find that the tissue is friable and does not repair well. The same principles of hygiene and suturing expertise should be followed. It is interesting that some mothers appear to have labial lacerations and that a rethinking of the need to suture may be required. Suturing in alternative positions, i.e. on birthing floor mattresses, takes a little learning. Cronk and Flint (1989, p.62) show how to suture in alternative positions.

Delay in placental delivery

The main thing about third-stage management is the requirement for great patience. If you have discussed physiological management with the mother she should also be aware that this may take up to two hours. Most mothers in my experience are content not to have syntometrine, and happy that I will only give an oxytocic drug if she starts to bleed. In other words I do not back out of physiological management and confuse the uterus by allowing it to start contracting and then add a new element, syntometrine. If the mother wishes to have syntometrine, I simply pull the plug, or ask her to leave the water immediately and give the drug as soon as possible. Its action is designed to stimulate a rapid contraction soon after newborn delivery, and thus initial placental bed size reduction.

A prerequisite to offering physiological third stage is that you are confident in undertaking this procedure, and that you believe that this woman is healthy and well. It is worth checking previous history and last haemoglobin check. I consider that when the woman has had a normal, non-interventionist first and second stage it is necessary to administer syntometrine routinely. It is worth remembering that oxytocic drugs were introduced in a very different era, when clients were neither well nourished nor screened and that labours were managed very differently.

Midwives' concerns about their own protection

As midwives we are well aware that we must take reasonable precautions to prevent danger to our mothers, but what about protecting ourselves? It has been suggested that midwives may suffer from back strain when undertaking waterbirths. Whilst it is true that the position for labour and delivery may be rather different I suspect that many of us have found ourselves delivering on the floor or in the toilet (wedged up against the wall)! So what lessons can be learnt from these encounters? I advise midwives to work out prior to their first waterbirth the position in which they will stand, sit or kneel and that you sort out what sort of supports you need. Cushions, beanbags and stools can all make it a more comfortable time, and will assist in supporting you and your back. Basic thoughts about posture can prevent problems later on. A word with your physiotherapy department could put a different viewpoint on positioning and height of tubs. More formal exercises are suggested by Balaskas and Gordon (1990, p.172–75). Precautions against cross-infection are dealt with in detail in Chapter Five.

Conclusion

It can be seen that many of these complications or problems could be overcome before they even occur. To anticipate and refer when appropriate is the art and skill of midwifery.

Overcoming difficulties starts by identifying your 'worst scenario' and what problems this will produce. My own concern is related to delay in the placental delivery, other colleagues have different concerns. As midwives we are all skilled enough to work through what is and what is not possible or practical in water. Skill-sharing with peers enables us to learn from our own, and others' clinical experiences. Whether the skill-sharing is formal through debriefing sessions, or individual in your reflective diary, the value of this learning curve should not be underestimated.

Ongoing education through workshops and literature reviews all assist midwives in developing their clinical and theoretical skills. Educational sessions may be organised locally, or you could be the light that sparks the fire within the hospital or community.

Forge links with other midwives and mothers who are involved with water labour/births, or companies who are hiring out water tubs. International links are possible through a variety of contact addresses, which are available at the end of this book.

CHAPTER ELEVEN

Midwives' education

Throughout this book I have highlighted and alluded to the fact that although waterbirths are seen as normal midwifery practice by our professional organisations, we have a responsibility to ensure that we acquire and maintain the necessary skills.

If midwives are not provided with both formal and informal education, a supportive environment within which to practice and a clinical audit that reflects their practice, it will be difficult for them to develop a waterbirthing service. I believe that it does not matter where or how midwives work – in hospital, home, teams, group practices or independently – we all have the same responsibility to ourselves and our clients. Within the most supportive frameworks for care, waterbirthing midwives have developed services that truly reflect women's choices and have audited their practice to enhance the body of evidence in practice.

In my experience there is often a willingness to develop a service in hospital or the home, but because of either professional or financial constraints this has not been able to grow. I would like to use this chapter to suggest some ways that midwives may be able to support their practice through education (both formal and informal) and gain experience prior to their first waterbirth.

With the introduction of PREP (Post Registration Education and Practice) midwives are able to gear their educational requirements more to their particular needs. It also encourages a more lateral development of learning opportunities, which assists midwives in gaining confidence and competence (in this scenario, in using water).

Formal education

Review code of practice

As with any new or ongoing skill, midwives need to ensure that they regularly review their rules and code of practice. The code is very clear regarding our responsibility to ensure that we are competent in skills acquired during training or those we have learnt following registration, and that we are accountable to ensure that through a variety of learning methods these skills are maintained.

I have described below some ideas for education opportunities, which could constitute learning on waterbirths. The main issue is often more to do with access to learning rather than the willingness to undertake the education. We have a responsibilty to attend, but our employer and supervisors also have a responsibilty to ensure that such opportunities are available to us.

Attendance at lectures/study days and in-house educational sessions

These may be run by the local educational provider or commercial organisations. Whichever you attend will depend on your own objectives and needs, the requirements from your Trust or Supervisor of Midwives and will have the ability to fulfil your code of practice and PREP.

Sessions at local level, as part of ongoing education

It may be useful to set up several of these, including:

- back to basics session – overview of waterbirths
- waterbirth update – new or interesting issues
- hot gossip – media or professional concerns (HIV testing or poor neonatal outcomes)
- dry run (see below)
- waterbirth audits.

Each unit and individual midwife will have their own agenda of formal education. However, as with any education it should be accessible and relevant to local needs. It should involve managers, the supervisor of midwives and other professionals within your organisation.

This link can be vital in sharing information and gaining assistance in situations in which other professionals have clinical expertise (i.e. lifting and handling, or infection control).

Set up guidelines

There are very good local and national guidelines which you can use as a base for new practitioners. They should be referenced and updated regularly. The guidelines should be set up by a multi-professional group, and should be made available to all new staff and parents.

Informal education

Networking with colleagues

This may be undertaken by use of the Internet and a website or an email address, or just good old-fashioned pen and paper. It is really important that we network with other professionals and midwives who are undertaking waterbirths. We can share knowledge and resources, and when untoward events occur we have easy and quick access to others who may have already encountered this event.

Specialist interest groups and individuals

These often exist, and the Royal Colleges and MIDIRS may act as a resource. Internationally, a small body of dedicated people are networking in practice, information sharing and audit. One such organisation is Global Maternal Child Health at www.waterbirth.org.

Reviewing fringe issues

It often becomes the case that when a unit begins to offer water labours/births, other practices are challenged. These fringe issues (routine CTGs, diet in labour, physiological third stage, routine ARM or vaginal examinations) may need to be reviewed. As all practice should be evidence-based, this challenge to accepted practice can often cause extra concerns. However, many of the fringe issues do have an impact on the way care is provided and may need to be addressed, often before water is introduced as a choice for women. The whole issue of challenging practice can in itself cause concern, and so this should always be undertaken in an open, reflective and supportive environment. When this is done I have found that many clinical issues can be freely discussed and if required amended, adapted or changed.

Literature search

Many organisations and libraries now have literature searches and bibliographies on waterbirth. A central accessible reference file is essential for midwives, so that they have access to literature and articles.

Some units have a noticeboard available containing new literature or changes to practice. Again the same principle exists; it should be accessible and up-to-date.

Set up a resource centre

Many units have benefited from setting up a resource centre containing information obtained about waterbirths. This can consist of literature, videos, books and any professional contacts. The main issue with any resource is that it is easily accessible and kept up-to-date. In my own unit we have a dedicated noticeboard for waterbirths on the labour ward, and all other information is kept by the practice and research midwife. Whilst this resource is in her office it has ensured that information does not get removed and is available for all staff, in addition to visitors and parents.

Local newsletter

This has been established by several units, both for mothers and professionals, to assist them in keeping up-to-date with new waterbirth issues. An existing hospital publication could be used, or midwives could be given the opportunity to design a newsletter that reflects local issues, whilst acting as a point of reference.

Professional visits

These have, in my opinion, become a more popular method of obtaining information from other units. Over the years, I have taken every opportunity to meet and speak with colleagues who undertake water-births. I have incorporated visits to units in other countries with attendance at ICM conferences, where I quite naturally meet colleagues. I have always found other units very welcoming and open to discussion. Some units have become so popular that they now charge for visits. However, as communication with websites and email develops, this, hopefully, will make units more accessible to all.

Clinical observation

This type of learning opportunity may lead on from a professional visit. Many units offer clinical observation. Although this is not yet common in the UK, it has been my experience abroad, particularly in America. Local units may be willing for colleagues to act as birth companions to women, transferring care from your own unit. This is particularly important, as the issues of honorary contracts are not always easy to initiate. It is always worth investigating this option, if you, your employer and the other Trust are willing to negotiate for this type of observation.

If clinical observation is organised, it is vital that both a format and guidelines for the visit are recorded; this could then be used as a PREP learning opportunity and recorded in your portfolio.

It is also worth noting that just as with professional visits, units may charge for this observational visit (bear in mind that there are administrative issues and a commitment for staff to support any visitors). However, on a local level, I have always found colleagues very keen to 'skill-share' their experiences with new midwives, and I have known doctors and GPs to ask to attend (with the mother's permission). Learning from each other is surely the most rewarding part of our role.

Dry runs

Over the past few years I have found that it is vital to carry out 'dry runs' in the actual setting of where the birthing pools are to be used. During the session that I undertake, we discuss the practical aspects of where to place equipment, how to protect your back and any other health and safety concerns (lifting and handling, water spillages).

Experiment with any existing lifting and handling equipment on a regular basis, and be aware of any new equipment or changes to the room.

In twelve years of using this method, I have never heard of any staff facing the problem of failing to feel prepared for the practical side of room preparation. In this session I cover the midwives' 'worst scenario' (PPH, shoulder dystocia) and then discuss with them what can be done practically, physiologically and safely. Please review Chapter Ten ' What if...' as a back up to this aspect of clinical preparation.

Design audit forms

If we are to provide evidence for our practice it is vital that we promote the use of audit in water labours/births. A sample audit form has been included in Chapter Nine and this could be used as a basis for local audit requirements. It is important, however, that any audit reflects local need and the requests from practitioners within your own sphere of practice. These audit forms may require ethical or audit department approval, and should maintain client confidentiality.

Some units have the benefit of computerised records, which can lend themselves to audits; however, these again, require a knowledge of IT skills, need to reflect local need, maintain confidentiality and UKCC standards on record keeping. Audits should be regularly presented at local level to ensure that information is up-to-date, accessible and utilised by midwives actually in clinical practice.

Waterbirth quiz

One very valuable learning opportunity can be gained through shared experiences with women who may not fall within a 'normality' criteria. At Maidstone Hospital, Kent, the unit has designed a quiz, which is given to new staff when they join the unit and is updated as other clients express an interest in using water for labour/delivery.

MIDWIFERY LEARNING THROUGH SHARED QUIZ

- Which of the following women would you feel happy to offer a water labour or birth to?

- Which would you offer a dry land rather than water third stage to?

- Which do you feel should not use water at all and why?

- Use your clinical judgement and experience, review local guidelines and ask your colleagues' opinions.

In some cases there is not always a definitive answer.

	Waterlabour	Waterbirth	Dry land 3rd stage	Do not use water	Reasons
IVF conception					
Previous LSCS					
Previous NND/SB					
Grand Multip					
Maternal age <15 years					
Maternal age >45 years					
Maternal weight >15 stone					
Deaf client					
Client with limited English					
Twins					
Breech					
Gestational diabetic					
Epileptic					
DVT on pill					
Myomectomy					

Cone biopsy					
Haemoglobinopathies					
Hb <10					
Maternal antibodies					
APH at 22/40					
Pregnancy induced hypertension					
Pre Eclampsia					
Maternal cardiac abnormality					
PRoM >24 hours					
Post mature >42/40					
Pethidine <4 hours ago					
Previous long labour					
Previous rapid delivery					
Previous third degree tear					
Previous episiotomy					
Previous retained placenta					
Previous Strep. B. carrier					
Known HIV/Hepatitis mother					
Vulval varicosities					
Vulval warts					
Previous history of herpes					
Symphysis pubis dysfunction					
Hip arthritis					
Umbilical hernia					
Maternal venflon in situ					
Baby with TOF					
Baby with dilated renal pelves					
Baby with kidney disease					

All of the above cases are based on women who have approached the author over the past eleven years.

Assumptions are made about the advantages and disadvantages of using water.

These summaries could be used as discussion points for midwives at the start of their education, as they raise many of the concerns that midwives and other staff highlight at the beginning of waterbirth practice.

Advantages of using water

The advantages of using water are as follows:

- Mother's choice and control in mode of labour/delivery
- Increases acceptance of 'normal' midwifery practice/challenges accepted/traditional patterns and type of care
- Regain 'traditional' skills
- Pleasant/relaxing environment
- Drug-free environment
- Non-interventionalist approach to care
- Attracts clients to unit for delivery
- Attracts staff recruitment
- Good PR for unit
- Increased parental/midwife liaison
- Income generation (pool hire)
- (Arguably) Improved clinical outcomes – Apgar scores/length of labour/perineal trauma
- (Arguably) Improved long term neonatal development.

Disadvantages of using water

The disadvantages of using water are as follows:

- Cost of tub or facilities may be prohibitive
- Client selection – defining normality may be dependent on the unit or midwife
- Clinical issues – need to record and review any negative outcomes
- Physiological issues – need to review newborn and maternal physiology
- Midwife education – access to appropriate education and resources
- Discrepancy between Trust policy and midwifery practice
- Standard setting – learning curve for midwives, need for appropriate support
- Access to appropriate equipment
- Seen as 'elitist' – may not be available to all women, depending on the midwives on duty or the locality of the unit
- Midwife outcomes – personal philosophy to care and injury

Education of Midwives is essential. It ensures that we maintain our skills, develop new areas of practice and provide our clients with the highest standard of care. Since undertaking my first waterbirth in 1989 I have embarked on a path of continuing and lifelong learning. I have never ceased to be amazed by this true path of discovery. I hope that as you conclude with the final chapter, this book will have triggered within you the same enthusiasm for learning.

Good luck on your voyage of discovery.

CHAPTER TWELVE

The final word

This last chapter is for all the other health professionals, and some of Maidstone parents. These accounts explain their own viewpoints, and share with you their experiences and feelings during the past eleven years of using water in practice at Maidstone.

John – the senior estates officer

Our first problem was to find a suitable bath manufactured in glass fibre, which would be large enough and comfortable enough for a mother to give birth in. A local manufacturer was found, and on our second project became involved in the design stage. A suitable room had then to be found on the delivery suite, since the volume and weight of the tub would mean that careful consideration needed to be given to the floors and access to water/drainage systems. The original tub weighed 1,292lb, and when the second larger one was installed the total estimated weight was 1,870lb.

When the original tub was delivered to the site we involved staff from maternity, to see how the layout of the room would fit in with the tub size. Carpenters and plumbers then installed the tub, with constant consultation from all those involved. Issues of lighting and ventilation needed to be tackled; the bright fluorescent lights were removed and spotlights on dimmer switches were installed. It also became apparent that adequate ventilation was needed, and an extractor fan was installed with the second tub. One safety factor was discussed with staff, and with agreement conventional bath taps were installed in both the Lagoon and Marine rooms, with no reported instances of client scalding.

The tubs have not caused any problems with ongoing maintenance, apart from a few tap washer changes, and one small chip in the tub which was dealt with by the manufacturer (we think some heavy object was dropped into the tub and that it was not a design problem).

Dawn – a mother

When I suggested to my husband Mike that I wished to have a waterbirth, my idea wasn't brushed aside as being a whim. He immediately sat down and started to design our own water tub (he's the supportive type).

I tried to do some more research into the concept of waterbirths, but there was little written about the subject – all I had to go on was my memory of a Russian waterbirth shown on television some years before. I approached my midwife Linda to see if there was any possibility that my wishes could be achieved. She brought in Dianne who had expressed great interest in what I was planning. After much discussion and negotiation (and I suspect red tape cutting), the water tub was available for use on the maternity unit.

On D-day I went into labour earlier than expected. My husband went to the hospital and set up the tub with Dianne. I was finding things difficult to cope with by the time I arrived at the hospital and was nearly ready to have all the pain relief going and not the tranquil, non-intervention, natural birth I'd planned. I got into the water as soon as possible. What bliss, my pain ceased, I was back in control and I started to drift. As I fancied the idyllic surroundings of a blue lagoon on a tropical island, I was able to ride out the wave of pain. I was able to see as my daughter was born, eyes closed and pink. She was gently lifted on to my chest and immediately started to breastfeed. No words can describe the joy I felt at that moment.

The experience was totally relaxed and wonderful – I'm so pleased that in our own way we've been able to make it possible for other mothers to experience this type of birth.

Linda – a community midwife and aquanatal teacher

As a midwife attached to a unit which practices water labour and birth (and having been involved from the beginning with this service), the idea of aquanatal appeared a natural progression. Initially we were guided by a physiotherapist, but as demand increased and the service developed, it became obvious that in order to offer the best service we would need to undertake an aerobic and subsequently a specific aquafit course for midwives. It is important that the teachers are qualified, and it is obviously a benefit that we are also midwives. Each woman is carefully screened before each class, to exclude certain conditions, eg. pre-eclampsia.

As the women gain confidence in themselves and lose their self-consciousness, we as midwives are able to feel rewarded that the class is giving tremendous support. The social aspect of the class is important, as the women get to know others in a similar position. Their reaction after the class is usually to remark on how good it is to be able to exercise in water, with no adverse effects for the baby. The suppleness and buoyancy assist the mothers in undertaking exercises that would not be possible on dry land. My enthusiasm stems from their enthusiasm, and as I keep the classes light and full of laughter, I am rewarded in return with their laughter.

Kim – a mother

The first I heard of waterbirths was when the Lagoon room opened at the hospital and it appeared in the local paper. As soon as I found out that I was pregnant, I did the usual thing of buying every magazine I could lay my hands on. Waterbirths were always spoken about (although usually only a small paragraph). Maidstone was mentioned in these texts as a 'pioneering unit' and I was pleased to be booked into such a hospital.

When I was about 7 months pregnant, I bought the Babywatching video by Desmond Morris. I was so impressed about the reasoning behind waterbirths as a natural concept to birth that I decided this was definitely for me. I might add that I don't see myself as being particularly brave with regard to pain – I hate going to the dentist!

The day I went into labour was nothing short of normal. I thought this couldn't be labour, it wasn't hurting enough. I eventually went into the hospital and found that I was already 4-5cm dilated. The midwives swapped over as I needed one who had experience and was to share the delivery with some other midwives (I was asked if I minded and I didn't). The baby's heartbeat and water temperature were constantly checked, and I had three midwives with me all the time. I was able to concentrate on what my body wanted to do, as the room was quiet most of the time. My daughter was born and brought up on to my stomach. She didn't cry at first and just snuggled up to me. My husband was with me throughout the labour and delivery, and gave me encouragement during the birth. He also had time to cuddle our daughter while I delivered the placenta.

I really enjoyed having my baby, and although I had a few stitches I felt I could have gone through the delivery again the next day. I am now 6 months pregnant with our second child, and am looking forward to the delivery. I still feel so relaxed and confident about labour and birth, that even if the water was not available I wouldn't mind.

Phyllis – an infection control nurse

When it was suggested that a specially designed, plumbed-in birthing bath should be installed in our obstetric department, I have to admit that I was filled with trepidation. Having trained as a midwife and then, following a break in service, as an infection control nurse, my first thoughts were regarding the infection risks. It is well-known that Gram-negative micro-organisms thrive in a warm, moist environment; the pathogen *Pseudomonas aeroginosa* has been isolated from waste pipes and drain outlets and Legionellae have been known to exist in shower heads. Also, what about the many potentially pathogenic micro-organisms which may be carried on the skin of the mother and attending midwives?

Discussions were held with the consultant medical microbiologist who shared my fears. However, it was decided that the infection risks could be markedly reduced by careful planning of the environment and by drawing up a policy which would have to be strictly observed before, during and after an underwater delivery. This included the choice of a very simple birthing bath, with no nooks and crannies to harbour bacteria and no whirlpool, heater or pump. Impeccable personal hygiene of both mother and midwife was demanded. A strict domestic hygiene protocol and on-going maintenance programme was set up to ensure that fixtures, fittings and plumbing remained in good order.

Some eleven years later, it would appear that our strategy has been successful for there have been no infections of mothers or babies directly linked to an underwater delivery. This must be entirely due to the diligence of a dedicated team who are totally committed to providing a safe environment, skilled practice and a happy delivery for mother and baby.

Lyndsey – a community midwife

Having run the gauntlet of change during the last 25 years of midwifery, it was with some diffidence that I entertained the idea of birth underwater. Publicity bred curiosity, clients expressed interest, and I felt compelled to learn more.

When a labouring woman slips gratefully into warm water and comments 'this is the best thing since sliced bread', you watch her visibly relax before your eyes, the only evidence of a contraction is her gentle rhythmic breathing, and the stirring of her swollen abdomen underneath the water as an aid during labour.

To witness your first birth underwater is an unnerving experience; after years of controlling the head, a hands off technique and minimal intervention comes hard! A gentle murmur from a baby in its mothers arms is still a sight that reminds me how privileged we are to share the birth of a couple's baby. Now after several years doing water deliveries, the privilege remains. For those mothers who enjoy the comfort of the water, I feel the advantages of its use far outweigh any potential disadvantages. As an analgesic, muscle relaxant, stress alleviator, hypotensive agent and diuretic, water does an admirable job. Perineal trauma appears to be minimal, fetal distress rare, labours are enhanced and shortened – eliminating maternal distress, ketosis and uterine inertia.

For the motivated women the water offers her the chance to fulfil her expectations. It gives her freedom of movement, non-invasive pain relief and control over her labour, that both she and her partner can fully appreciate.

As a community midwife I have found the use of water at home offers an aid to a peaceful and speedy first stage – to the point that labour is so fast that you should be prepared to deliver at home! Fears of the unknown are understandable - shoulder dystocia and water inhalation are two. A mother in the water is far more able to stand up or squat to assist shoulder delivery, and regular checks on water temperature should assist in avoiding water inhalation.

Finally, a waterbirth at home is one of the most beautiful experiences I have ever had.

Joanne – a mother

In my experience things rarely go to plan. I had decided not to write a formal birth plan, but rather leave my options open, having some idea of what I'd like to try if all was going well. As anticipated things did not go quite to plan. I was booked for induction the following week, so my husband decided to travel to Scotland to complete some work prior to the birth of our baby.

'What are you doing today?' he'd asked before leaving on his mammoth journey at 4.30am. 'Having a baby!' I'd replied jokingly. This couldn't have been closer to the truth.

Towards lunchtime I had a couple of 'period-like' pains. Suspecting that the pains were psychological due to my husband's absence, I swam for one mile as usual. Later in the day, the pains were becoming stronger and more regular. I contacted the hospital and went in for an examination. Yes, I was in labour! My husband was promptly instructed to begin his return journey.

During early labour I was able to use breathing techniques to cope with the contractions. I explained to the midwife that if all was going well, I would like to try TENS and water for pain relief when the contractions became stronger (but not at the same time!). I also added that I would prefer a dry land delivery. The TENS was very effective for some considerable time. However with the contractions becoming much stronger my midwife suggested that if I wished to try the water, now would be a good time. So I did. I have to admit that the thought of parting with the TENS machine at this point made me more than a little apprehensive. My midwife reassured me that I could have the TENS machine back on within a couple of minutes if I did not like the water.

It was amazing. I found the water so soothing, relaxing and a really effective form of pain relief when combined with relaxation breathing techniques. The 'Marine' birthing room looked lovely with a mural of dolphins and fish on the walls. These pictures combined with my excellent midwife really helped me to concentrate my mind and ride through those contractions. The time passed very quickly, and I progressed very well (almost too well, as my husband arrived only 20 minutes before our daughter was born).

The time had come for me to leave the pool if I wanted to deliver on dry land as I had intended, but the water was so relaxing that I couldn't even consider getting out. I decided therefore to have a waterbirth. From starting pushing our daughter was born within 20 minutes, which is certainly not long for a first baby. The whole of my labour had lasted less than eight hours. My husband and I were both very impressed with the labour and delivery. I'm sure we'll never forget the wonderful experience as our daughter Kate emerged on to my stomach from under the water, wide-eyed and ready washed!

Before having Kate I had not really considered waterbirth, as I had wrongly assumed it to be a messy and a 'way out' option.

Both my husband and I are now totally converted to waterbirth. I would love to have one again, and only hope that it will be as enjoyable the next time round. Now 12 weeks on, I am still talking about how wonderful the birth was. Friends in other parts of the country are quite envious of my labour and birthing experiences. Our water baby Kate, also seems to have had a very positive experience. She has a lovely temperament and always enjoys her bath, crying only when we take her out!

Alan – an obstetrician

The theoretical basis for waterbirths is still uncertain. As an obstetrician I feel happy to have the facility available and pleased that the body of evidence for safety is growing. But for my own wife I would not yet be quite sure. However where theoretical basis for birth under water is not clear, a mass of empirical data may well resolve the question. That position appears to be approaching regarding waterbirths.

When used in the first stage of labour there seems to be little doubt that warm water is preferable to drugs, providing the water temperature is well controlled and infection is excluded.

With the influx of any new technique there is undoubtedly an enthusiasm factor. Epidurals were introduced and performed by myself some 20 years ago, and they were rapturously received partly because they were new and fervently performed. With time they became part of the routine and part of client expectations. The same could happen with waterbirths.

Patient choice is an excellent entity and to be encouraged, but one must always bear in mind the medico-legal situation. It is in the interests of all concerned with waterbirths to see that the protocols are strict and audit is clear. Happily midwives are much better at setting protocols and monitoring cases than doctors are.

Denise – a mother

I wanted to have a waterbirth with my daughter in 1991 but didn't want to feel 'she just wants to be different'! I ended up with a 24½ hour labour and taking everything to ease the pain.

When I was expecting my son in 1993, I definitely wanted to have a waterbirth. I felt it was an experience I wanted to endure. However, my husband was nervous. What if he drowns, or there is a problem? These fears and questions were all answered by our community midwife.

A friend who had given birth to her third daughter in the bath a year before told me of how she experienced less pain and a truly easier delivery. I thought, it can't be that different. How wrong I was to be.

I was in fact induced. First stage labour pains lasted 6 hours 45 minutes until I was 7cm dilated without using any painkillers, only breathing techniques and my husband frantically rubbing my back. It was then decided that I was ready to get into the bath. I wondered how many more hours! As I lowered myself into the bath I couldn't believe how warm, comfortable and calm I was. I nervously awaited the next painful contraction in my back, gritted my teeth and held on to my husband's hand, hard. It came and I would honestly say it seemed to be half the pain and seemed to be over quicker. On I went for 11 minutes, calm and totally in control. With soft lights and quiet music, I gave birth to my son. It was wonderful. I had only been in the bath for 21 minutes and had done so much. My son was calmly lifted slowly from the water on to my chest. As he looked up at me, we cried with joy and relief that it had gone so well. He was so calm, I think he could have enjoyed it as well. He was given to my husband for a cuddle and I got out of the bath for the third stage.

I had no grazes, stitches or inflammation and still seemed to have so much energy. I felt so well, other mothers on my ward were amazed at my story. My son has no fear of water and still at one year old loves a good splash in the bath.

I would give other parents encouragement to have a waterbirth, I'm sure that it would be an experience they would never forget.

Mike – the purchaser

A purchaser's viewpoint will concentrate on benefits, costs and quality. Both benefits and costs carry a lot of meaning, so what do they imply?

Healthcare purchasers, whether a health authority or fund holders, want to purchase effective healthcare; they will also be committed to implementing *Changing Childbirth*. They will, through service specifications and contracts want to ensure that the woman can exercise informed choice. This may include the choice of various methods of pain relief, labour position and delivery mode and the water bath may be the woman's choice for each of these. Other benefits may include a shortened labour, less analgesia and a more contented relaxed mother.

The purchasers will also want to be informed and assured about all the possible costs. These obviously include direct monetary costs associated with water facilities and staffing, both when all goes well and perhaps, more so, if it doesn't. Safety is therefore of high importance both for mother and baby directly, but also in the context of possible litigation.

Where any procedure, whether truly new or reintroduced, is involved purchasers will want evidence of the effectiveness, i.e. proof of the claimed benefits, and safety. Increasingly from now on they will want to see research evidence, and the involvement of participating units, staff and clients in research, data collection and analysis. Finally, purchasers are increasingly requiring healthcare quality assurance which implies acceptance of all of the above points and ongoing clinical audit and use of consumer satisfaction surveys.

Beverley – a mother

Even before being pregnant I was fascinated and intrigued by people's accounts of waterbirth. So when I found out that I was expecting a baby, using water in some way was definitely on my mind.

My local community midwife was able to answer my queries and showed pictures of waterbirths that she had attended. As time went by I gradually shifted from wanting to labour in water to wanting to actually give birth in water.

My husband was happy about this as long as he didn't have to strip off and join me! I practised being in water at home – in the bath at least once a day, sometimes using essential oils. I used to trickle water over my bump and the baby would respond. They were special times in the bath – me and my bump.

On my due date my blood pressure shot up and there it stayed. After three pessaries I was still not in labour. Eventually my waters were broken and with my blood pressure now settling, a different midwife (due to a shift change) asked if I would like to use the water. I got into the bath and lay on my front with my chest, arms and head on a ledge in the bath. The relief was incredible and instant, the room was quiet and warm (almost muted) and incredibly soothing. After three contractions in the water I had the most incredible urge to push. I was petrified as I thought I was only 5cm dilated. My husband went rushing out to fetch the midwife and as she came in I can remember saying to her 'whatever you say I'm going to push'. My son was delivered with the next contraction, only 14 minutes after I got into the water.

Jack was calm and content and didn't cry the whole time we were in hospital. He still enjoys his bath and now at 6 months goes swimming and does not seem to mind going under water.

My husband was fascinated by being able to see our baby's face perfectly under water. I would definitely have another waterbirth as long as circumstances allow, and feel that it was due to the water that my labour and birth were not traumatic to me, my husband or our son.

Mary – Supervisor of Midwives

Creating an environment conducive to high standards and professional practice, providing support and acting as an advocate for both mothers and midwives, are high on the agenda of the Supervisors of Midwives within the current NHS environment. Central to the role of supervision is the safety and wellbeing of mothers and babies. However, as a Supervisor working in a unit which practices waterbirth, I firmly believe we need to also offer a supportive network to midwives.

The practice of waterbirth was a new concept to us all in 1987. As we already worked in a proactive unit the way was paved for practitioners who wished to react to these requests with enthusiasm and vision. The enabling process began with regular meetings, 'brainstorming', research and facilitation of practice development. As we were all students on this learning curve, we respected and supported each other. Clearly

Responsibilities and Sphere of Practice (Rule 40), now aids midwives in this process. Research, education and development of new skills is each midwife's own responsibility, but the process of supervision involves ensuring that a safe level of competence and confidence has been reached.

When practice requires the acquisition of new skills, supervisors should be sought and consulted with about these new skills. As mothers become more assertive, midwives, too, need to feel competent and confident, in order to be able to empower women.

A continuous programme of skill-sharing, peer support and education is required. I also firmly believe that the role of the supervisors is to support midwives if they have a dilemma with delivering women in water. Many colleagues have been trained in the 'medical model' where delivery is only normal in retrospect.

It is important to agree local guidelines and standards, and to draw these up with the local supervisor and other personnel who are likely to be involved. They should be available to all midwives within their supervisory jurisdiction. The importance of record keeping cannot be stressed too strongly, writing notes contemporaneously will assist midwives in decision-making.

Waterbirth is seen as one mode of delivery within our unit, supported by the Trust and as supervisors we are keen to keep these deliveries in perspective. The objective of supervision is to initiate a positive, proactive approach, empowering midwives to enhance their practice and thus the quality of care.

Rachel – a mother

My first labour was over 20 hours long. I felt as though I was dying and had very negative feelings about the whole experience. The baby cried for the next 48 hours, between catnaps. I think it had been traumatic for him too.

My second labour was slow getting underway. I was sent up to the antenatal ward and when the contractions became businesslike, I asked to have a bath. It was a deep bath and I spent an hour humming my way through the contractions in a sort of dream. It was peaceful and private – just me and my husband, but with the security of a call button. When the pain became too great I was wheeled down to the labour ward for some gas and air, and found I was 8cm dilated. The second stage was straightforward, comparatively quick and I felt on cloud nine.

I read as much as I could on the subject of waterbirths. My GP told me that Maidstone was the place to go, and no sooner had I explained to my family and friends why I was going to Maidstone that the news reports about the dangers of waterbirth were broadcast. I decided that the risks (some hypothetical) were smaller than the overall risks involved in childbirth.

I did have a water labour, although I stood up for the delivery to utilise gravity. My feelings afterwards were those of feeling triumphant. The pregnancy had been hard work for all of us, but the positive birth experience and lovely natured baby made it all worthwhile. Although some of my dreams were not possible, like giving the first breastfeed in water, I know that under the circumstances I still had a wonderful delivery.

Keith – a researcher

The controversy surrounding the safety of waterbirth has abated in recent years, probably because no untoward events have occurred, or been reported since the problems encountered in 1993. A modest stream of articles has appeared in the professional press and the topic was discussed at the ICM in Manila early in 1999. From my own work I am conscious that we have not achieved any significant advances in the quality of evidence we are able to provide to clients, practitioners, managers and politicians regarding the effectiveness of waterbirth. This creates a feeling that waterbirth is 'tolerated' rather than greeted with enthusiasm. If it were possible to demonstrate the observed benefits 'scientifically' by means of the much-revered method of the randomised controlled trial, I am sure that professional attitudes would change swiftly and that this would lead to an increase in the number of waterbirths.

My strong belief in the individual mother's right to exercise as much personal choice as she wishes when giving birth – based on clinically-feasible options – has not changed. This stems from the belief that bringing a child into the world should be a fulfilling experience and not one of ritualised abuse. Given that western women tend to have few children, the opportunities for them to have such an experience are quite rare. It seems unethical to attempt to inveigle them into trial groups that will, in some cases, certainly result in them experiencing modes of delivery that are contrary to their preferences. However, if it is not possible to randomly allocate clients to the trial groups, the randomised controlled trial is effectively scuppered. The method is also compromised by the obvious inability to apply blinding techniques, since both the mothers and midwives will be fully aware of the allocated group in each case.

As I mentioned in the first edition of this book, there seems to exist both a need and an opportunity to carry out research using mixed methods, some quantitative, other qualitative. Properly-conducted studies could bring about an understanding of the respective benefits and disadvantages of different birthing modes that is broader, richer and altogether more useful than the 'safety' and 'clinical' issues that have been the subject of much comment in the literature to date.

Rob – a father

Like most partners I wanted only what was best for my wife and the baby. Remembering how tense the hospital birth of my daughter, Chelsey, had been, I was more than willing for the next baby to be born in water in the relaxed atmosphere of our home.

Originally we had wanted to put the pool upstairs so that it would be near the bathroom, but were advised by a structural engineer that the existing floor would not take the weight. The cost of reinforcing the floor would have come to several thousand pounds, so we decided to put the pool downstairs. When I started assembling the pool it seemed awfully small. I don't know what I had expected, maybe something that one could stretch out in like the birthing tub we had seen at Maidstone hospital. But in retrospect I think the size was just right.

The thing that sticks most in my memory was how calm and peaceful the labour was compared to the hospital birth of Chelsey. This time there were no shift changes, no hospital rules, just the familiar environment of our own home. Chelsey, now four years old, was able to come and go as she pleased, and even got in the tub with Lauri for a while. She remembers now, a year later, how she helped rub her mummy's back and how useful that made her feel.

After the delivery of our son, the pain all forgotten, Lauri took him in her arms and cuddled him. I felt relief. It was over and we had a beautiful, healthy son. This time the labour and delivery had been a far more calm experience.

Morag – a home waterbirth mother

The contractions I had when I got out of the water were distinctly more painful than in the water, and I can imagine they would have caused me to tense up quite early on, thus making labour more painful, if I had laboured without water.

The delivery itself took place in the pool, and was an amazing calm moment. The baby came down the birth canal so fast, the midwife was still putting her gloves on in readiness for when his head appeared! Although we seemed to wait ages for his body to come out, we were calm because we had been warned in advance that this might happen, and as far as the baby was concerned, the pool was simply an extension of the womb. Our two midwives were very calm and reassuring. A very surreal experience! My baby was extremely calm and alert right from the moment that he came out of the water, and has stayed that way since.

Sarah – a midwife

After several years of wanting to undertake a waterbirth, and many labours later, my dream came true. I had witnessed two home waterbirths as a student and been second midwife at a few hospital waterbirths, so I knew the principles, but was 'itching' to put them into practice.

When the opportunity arose to transfer Stephanie to the labour ward, I jumped at the chance! This was her first baby and she and her husband had planned for a water labour and delivery. They were both well informed, having attended the 'Waterbirth evening', facilitated by Dianne.

Labour progressed normally. After being in the water only a short time Stephanie wanted to push. Nature took its course and the water visibly relaxed Stephanie and seemed to enable her body to be effective. She pushed involuntarily and it soon became obvious that the baby was about to be born. The desire to put my hands down and support the baby was almost overwhelming, but I managed to resist! As the baby was born, I gently lifted her into the waiting arms of her mother. A more gentle birth I find hard to imagine.

I have to say that the support from the midwifery sister on duty at the time further enhanced my confidence and now I am looking forward to my next waterbirth.

Jayn – a waterbirth mother and waterbirthing services owner

When I became preganant with Nathan in 1988 I was 34, unfit and overweight. However, I knew the birth was going to be one of the most important experiences of my life so I looked into everything really carefully, especially as this was my first baby. I saw a documentary on television of a waterbirth at home and read a newspaper article about Sheila Kitzinger's daughter, Tess, giving birth at home in water. I decided to opt for a waterbirth at home, with the option of going into hospital if I needed to for medical reasons, or if I felt I could not cope at home. My midwife had attended women labouring in water and supported me in my decision.

After the birth of Nathan, little did I realise that I was one of the first women in the UK to give birth in water. Because of the media coverage during my pregnancy and the fact that my midwife had attended several women labouring in water, I thought that this was quite a usual way to labour and give birth.

I set up Splashdown – a waterbirthing service – with two pools initially, and now have pools all over the UK. We have helped several thousand women to use water pools over the past eleven years and our expansion is continuing with midwives' study days and practical support.

Gill – clinical risk manager

The main principle of risk management within midwifery is to ensure safe delivery and up-to-date evidence-based care to all mothers and babies. Within the context of waterbirths this will come under two main areas, namely, clinical and environmental.

- *Clinical.* It is important that up-to-date, regularly-reviewed guidelines are available and that both the midwives and women requesting waterbirths are familiar with them. Women need to understand that if they are asked to leave the pool they should do so for their own or their baby's wellbeing. Midwives who undertake waterbirths should be competent to do so, or be supervised by someone who is. It is essential that adequate education is given as required.

- *Environmental.* Environmental risk management is particularly important in the home setting but applies equally in hospitals. It is important that the room that houses the birthing pool can bear its weight. Partners should be informed of their responsibilty towards filling/emptying or caring for the pool (this may vary between hospitals and home). Adequate lifting devices/or assistance from the partner should be made available. This should take into account local policies regarding manual handling.

Whichever element of risk management is examined, co-operation from the woman and her partner is essential They should be given full explanations and be encouraged to participate in a partnership approach to care, all of which will help to foster a supportive environment. Good communication channels are essential for optimum safety.

Alison – a mother

When I became pregnant with my first daughter, Madeline, I was determined to have as easy a delivery as possible. My mother had always told me that childbirth was a question of physical hard work and that the 'pain' was more the result of fear of the unknown and lack of knowledge. This led me to study the physiology of childbirth and to practice mind-over-matter meditation. I would strongly recommend anyone of like mind to read *Childbirth Without Fear* by Grantly Dick-Reid. Even though the book is now seriously out of date, the underlying ethos is still excellent. At the same time as mentally preparing myself, I got fit – swimming almost daily right up to the date of delivery. Apart from the fact that I love swimming, I was encouraged to do so because it is the best exercise in pregnancy. My great aunt who had been a keen swimmer, had two very quick and easy childbirths.

The notion of waterbirth came from a video borrowed from the NCT – the idea of being cocooned in warm water and feeling weightless during labour immediately appealed. A quick visit to the wonderful birthing pools at the hospital (more like en-suite bathrooms), with fish and octopus wall paintings confirmed my desire for a waterbirth.

The reality of Madeline's birth was better than I could have imagined. I spent the first stage labouring quietly in bed on my side in the adjacent room. Once I was sufficiently dilated and I started to feel the second stage urge to push, I asked to go into the pool. The warmth of the water was wonderfully comforting and it felt the most natural place in the world to be. I floated on my side for several contractions, puffing away the urge to push. Finally, when ready, I straddled the bath and pushed Madeline out. Her head appeared immediately and she was born within twenty minutes or so of my entering the pool.

My next two daughters Imogen and Jasmine were also born under water, each within twenty minutes of entering the water. Their births were even more straightforward. Knowing exactly what to expect, I got into the pool both times only when the urge to push came on, but unlike when giving birth to Madeline, I did not actually push. Instead I just floated on my side and gently let my body do all the work. As a result, I sustained no scratches or tears.

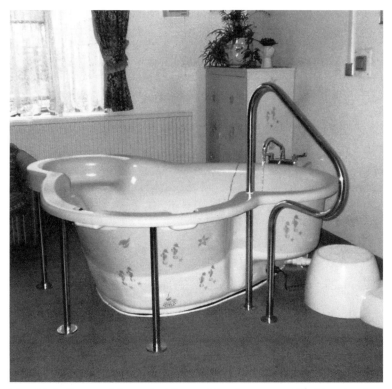

Fig. 12.1: Barratt Maternity Home, Northampton. Birthing Pool.

The atmosphere of all three births was so relaxed that my husband was able to take many photos of me and our daughters as they were born. He was particularly amazed to see the head and face of each child appear underwater and remain clearly in view between contractions. Each child will have her own birth album and hopefully this will encourage them to believe that childbirth is not necessarily something to be dreaded.

I am sure that I have been blessed with easy births, but I strongly believe that the preparation – mental and physical – did pay off. I may have a fourth child, and if I do, all being well, intend to go for water again.

Betty – a midwife

Our hospital had a limited waterbirth service, with women hiring their own pools and bringing them into the unit. This was not an ideal situation for women, midwives and the labour ward environment.

A small group of midwives at the hospital were interested in installing a pool on the labour ward. Having met Dianne at the International Waterbirth Conference and hearing about the waterbirth clinical placement her unit offered, I spent a week there in order to gain knowledge and confidence in using water in midwifery practice. The week was invaluable, giving access to clinical audit, review of world-wide literature, videos and having the opportunity to work and discuss with midwives experienced in waterbirths.

On my return I was convinced that we should have a pool within the unit. A midwifery-led initiative was set up, with a steering group and management support to search out information, pool availability, write guidelines and set up teaching sessions (to name but a few of our roles).

We have skill-shared between five unit midwives who already had waterbirth experience, provided cascaded learning, educational sessions (facilitated by Dianne) and joined the waterbirth audit.

The success of the project has resulted from excellent communication within the unit, committed, enthusiastic midwives and local publicity, with women writing about their birth experiences. Although there has been a lot of hard work and stress, the rewards have been considerable for both mothers and midwives.

And Lauri concludes...

At 3.50 I entered the water. It was wonderful. The contractions slowed a little giving me a very welcome break! My blood pressure also dropped to a more acceptable level. I spent most of the next few hours kneeling – supporting myself over the edge of the bath. The next few hours were filled with regular sips of cold water, listening to the baby's heart rate; water temperature checks; chocolate cake and contractions! Chelsey stayed in the room most of the time, supported by our friend Jo.

Rob says his overriding impression of the birth was one of real calm and peacefulness. I was overwhelmed by the normality of it all. And when I woke in the middle of the night to feel Chelsey crawling over me to gaze at her new brother, I knew we had definitely made the right choice.

Glossary

Acidosis	*A diminution of alkaline or increased acidity in the blood*
Adrenaline	*Hormone secreted by the medulla of the adrenal gland*
Adrenagenic	*The term applied to nerves that release the chemical transmitter noradrenaline*
Amniocentesis	*A surgical puncture through the amniotic sac to obtain a sample of amniotic fluid*
Antenatal	*The time period before birth*
Apgar score	*System devised to assess the condition of a baby during the first few minutes of life*
Artificial rupture	*Small hole pierced through the membranes with a small plastic clip*
Catecholamine	*A group of compounds that stimulate the sympathetic nervous system*
Caesarean	*An incision into the uterus to deliver the baby*
Cardiotocograph	*A graphical correlation between fetal heart rate pattern and uterine contractions*
Conception	*The fusion of spermatozoon and ovum*
Cortisol	*Naturally occurring hormone of the adrenal cortex*
Dysmenorrhoea	*Difficult or painful menstruation*
Dystocia	*Difficult or abnormal labour*
Endorphins	*Hormones that act at opiate sites and produce natural analgesia*
Entonox	*Nitrous oxide and oxygen 50:50 mix. Used as an inhalation analgesia*
Epidural	*Pain relief through injecting analgesic drugs into the epidural space in the spine*

Episiotomy	*An incision made into the thinned out perineal body to enlarge the vaginal orifice*
Ergometrine	*An alkaloid used to prevent or control postpartum bleeding*
Fetus	*The human embryo from the 5th week of pregnancy to the time of birth*
Glomerular filtration rate	*The amount of filtrate that flows out of the renal corpuscles of both kidneys*
Gravida	*A pregnant woman*
Haemoglobin	*Pigment contained in red blood cells, combines with oxygen to transport it to tissues*
Hepatitis	*Inflammation of the liver, usually due to a virus. Types include A, B and C*
HIV	*Human Immuno Deficiency Virus. A retro virus responsible for Acquired Immuno Deficiency Syndrome*
Homeopathy	*Use of substances (drugs) that treat like with like*
Hyperthermia	*Abnormally high body temperature*
Hypoglycaemia	*Abnormally low blood sugar*
Hypotension	*Blood pressure below the normal range*
Hypothermia	*A fall in body temperature to subnormal levels*
Hypoxia	*Diminished oxygen tension in the body tissues*
Inertia	*Inability of the uterine muscle to contract efficiently*
Intrapartum	*Within labour*
Ketosis	*Presence of ketones in the body, which occur when fat metabolism is disturbed as a result of carbohydrate lack*
Legionellae	*Gram negative bacillus often isolated from shower heads*
Liquor amnii	*The fluid which fills the amniotic sac surrounding the baby*
LSCS	*Lower Segment Caesarean Section*

Meconium	*Greenish black material present in the fetal intestinal tract*
Neonatal	*Pertaining to a newborn child*
Nuchal cord	*When the cord is round the baby's neck*
Oxytocin	*Hormone produced from the posterior pituitary gland, which stimulates uterine contractions*
Parity	*Having borne a baby*
Perineum	*Area extending from the pubic arch to the coccyx*
Peripheral resistance	*Refers to the resistance to the blood flow and the walls of the blood vessels*
Pethidine	*Narcotic injectable analgesia*
Placenta	*The 'afterbirth' which produces hormones and acts as a barrier during pregnancy*
Post partum	*After labour and delivery*
Pregnancy induced hypertension	*Raised blood pressure in pregnancy*
PREP	*Post Registration Education and Practice*
Prostin E	*Hormone pessary used to start labour*
Pseudomonas	*A bacillus normally found in the colon*
Rebirthing	*The art of transgressing to 'relive' birth*
Steroids	*Hormones with chemical structure of carbon and hydrogen eg. sex hormones*
Suture	*Stitches used to close a wound*
Syntocinon	*Synthetic form of hormone oxytocin*
Syntometrine	*Combined ergometrine/syntocinon used to assist delivery of the placenta*
Ultrasound	*Use of sound waves, to reflect between differing tissues to produce a picture*
VBAC	*Vaginal Birth After Caesarean*
Vernix	*The 'greasy' substance that covers the fetus in utero. Secreted from the sebaceous glands*

References

Aird A, Luckas M, Buckett WM *et al.* Effects of intrapartum hydrotherapy on labour related parameters. *Aust N Z J Obstet Gynaecol 1997*, 37(2): 137-42.

Alderdice F, Renfrew M, Marchant S, Ashurst H, Hughes P, Berridge G, Garcia J. Labour and birth in water in England and Wales. *BJM 1995*, 310: 837.

Alexander J, Levy V, Roch S. *Midwifery Practice: A research based approach.* London: Macmillan, 1993.

Anderson B, Gyhagan M, Nielson TF. Warm bath during labor: Effects on labour duration and maternal and fetal morbidity. *Am J Obstet Gynecol 1996*, 16: 326-30.

Austin T, Bridges N, Markiewicz M, Abrahamson E. Severe neonatal polycythaemia after third stage of labour underwater. *Lancet 1997*, 350: 1445.

Baddeley S. Aquanatal advantages. *Modern Midwife 1993* July/August: 16-8.

Baddeley S. Client health aquanatal classes. *ICM Conference Proceedings*. ICM: Manila, 1999.

Balaskas J, Gordon Y. *Waterbirth*. London: Unwin, 1990.

Barber P. *Who Cares for the Carers?* London: South Bank University, 1994.

Baum M. (1993). New approach for recruitment into randomised controlled trials. *Lancet 1993*, 341: 812-3.

Beech B. *Choosing a waterbirth.* London: AIMS, 1996.

Beech B. A visit to Vienna. *AIMS Journal 1996*, 8(1): 6-8.

Beech B. *Waterbirth Unplugged.* Manchester: Books for Midwives, 1996.

Blair Myers M. The lagoon room experience. *Nursing Times 1989*, 22nd November, Vol. 85.

Brook D. *Nature Birth*. Harmondsworth: Penguin, 1976.

Brown L. (1998). The tide has turned: Audit of water birth.' *BJM 1998*, 6(4): 236-43.

Brucker M. (1984). Nonpharmaceutical methods for relieving pain and discomfort during pregnancy. *MCN 1984*, 9: 390-4.

Burke H. (1985). The shock of birth. *Nursing Mirror 1985*, Sept 11th, 161: 41.

Burns E, Greenish K. Pooling information. *Nursing Times 1993*, February 24th, 89(8): 47-9.

Cain M. Taking to the water. *Midwives Chronicle 1992*, June, 148-9.

Cefalo RC, Andre U, Hellegers E. The effects on maternal hyperthermia on maternal and fetal cardiovascular and respiratory function. *Am J Obstet Gynecol 1978*, 131(6): 687-94.

Channel Four Television. *Brave New Babies: Learning before birth?* London: Channel 4, 1994.

Charles C. Fetal hyperthermic risk from warm water immersion. *BJM 1998*, 6(3): 152-6.

Clarke R. The last stand? *Nursing Times 1993*, 89(11).

Cluett E. Water, wait or augment? Randomised controlled trial of three management options for nulliparae with dystocia in the first stage of labour. *ICM Conference Proceedings*, ICM 1999.

Cochrane A, Callen K. *Beyond the Blue.* London: Bloomsbury, 1998.

Crawford JS. The phases and stages of labour. *MIDIRS Midwifery Digest 1987*, No 4, April.

Cronk M, Flint C. *Community Midwifery.* Oxford: Heinemann, 1989.

Crozier K, Sinclair M. Birth technology. *Midwives Journal 1999*, 2(5): 60-4.

Crumble A. American dream or American nightmare. *Nursing Standard 1993*, 7(19): 18-9.

Daniels K. Waterbirth. *Meditation 1988*, Winter, 36.

Daniels K. Waterbirth: The newest form of safe, gentle joyous birth. *J Nurse Midwifery 1989*, 34(4): 198.

Day M. Trust demands HIV test for pool births. *Nursing Times 1996*, 92(2): 9.

Department of Health. *Changing Childbirth: Report of the Expert Maternity Group.* London: HMSO, 1993.

Department of Health. *Reducing mother to child transmission of HIV infection in the UK.* London: HMSO, 1998.

Dick-Read, G. *Childbirth Without Fear.* New York: Perennial, 1953, reprinted 1984.

Doniec Ulman I, Kokot F, Wambach G, Drab M. Water immersion induced endocrine alterations in women with EPH gestosis. *Clin Nephrol 1987*, 28(2): 51-5.

Downe S, Kirkham M. *Politics and the Midwife*. London: South Bank University, 1993.

Editorial. Trust betrayed. *MIDIRS* 1994, 4(2): 132-3.

Eriksson M, Ladfors L, Mattson LA *et al*. Warm tub bath during labour. *Acta Obstet Gynecol Scand* 1996, 75(7): 642-4.

Eriksson M, Mattsson LA, Ladfors L. Early or late bath during the first stage of labour. *Midwifery* 1997, 13: 146-8.

Falconer AD, Powles AB. Plasma noradrenaline levels during labour. *Anaesthesia* 1982, 37: 416-20.

Farnworth J. Water play. *Parents* 1990, March: 58-60.

Flint C. Objections overruled? *Nursing Times*, 1986 April 2nd, 22.

Forde C, Creighton S, Batty A, Hawdon J, Summers-Ma S, Ridgway G. Labour and delivery in the birthing pool. *BJM* 1999, 7(3): 165-71.

Ford L, Garland D. An aqua birth concept. *Midwives Chronicle* 1989, July: 232-4.

Fox A. Midwife's a dolphin. *News of the World*, 30th August 1992, 16.

Garcia J, Redshaw M, Fitzsimmons B, Keene J. *First Class Delivery*. Abingdon: Audit Commission, 1998.

Garland D, Jones K. (1994). Waterbirth, 'first stage': Immersion or non immersion? *BJM* 1994, 2(3): 113-20.

Garland D, Jones K. Waterbirth: Updating the evidence. *BJM* 1997, 5(6): 368-73.

Gibb D. *A Practical Guide To Labour Management*. Oxford: Blackwell Scientific, 1988.

Gibb D, Arulkumaran S. *Fetal Monitoring In Practice*. Oxford: Butterworth Heinemann, 1992.

Gilbert RE, Tookey PA. Perinatal mortality and morbidity among babies delivered in water: Surveillance study and postal survey. *BMJ* 1999, 21st August, 319: 483-7.

Gillot de Vries F, Wesel S, Busine A, Adler A, Camus M, Patesson R, Gillard C. Influence of a bath during labor on the experience of maternity. *Pre and Perinatal Psychology* 1987, 1(4): 297-302.

Goodlin RC, Hoffmann KLE, Williams NE, Buchan P. Shoulder out, immersion in. *J Perinat Med* 1984, 12: 173-7.

Gradert Y, Hertel J, Lenstrup C, Bach FW, Christensen NJ, Roseno H. Warm tub during labor. *Acta Obstet Gynecol Scand* 1987, 66: 681-3.

Gyte G. The significance of blood loss at delivery. *MIDIRS Midwifery Digest*, 1992, 2: 1.

Halksworth G. *Aquanatal Exercises*. Manchester: Books for Midwives, 1994.

Hall SM, Holloway IM. Staying in control: Women's experiences of labour in water. *Midwifery* 1998, 14: 30-6.

Hamed H, Griffin CA, Mackinney LG, Sugiaka K. Role of caratoid chemoreceptors in the initiation of effective breathing of the lamb at term. *Paediatrics 1967*, 39(3): 329-36.

Harper B. Waterbirth international. *MIDIRS Midwifery Digest* 1990, 13, April.

Harper B. *Gentle Birth Choices*. Vermont, USA: Healing Arts Press, 1994.

Hawkins S. Water vs conventional births: Infection rates compared. *Nursing Times* 1995, 91(11): 38-40.

Health and Safety Executive. Control of substances hazardous to health. COSHH Regulations. London, 1999.

Hilson GRF. The real dangers of waterbabies. *Guardian*, 29th July 1994.

Hlavackova J. Alternativi porod. Baraka. *Leto* 1998, 50-7.

House of Commons Health Committee. *Maternity Services*. London: HMSO, 1992.

Hughes H. *Prenatal Water Workout Book*. New York: Avery Group, 1989.

Hughes R. The water babies. *Parents*, April 1989.

Huntingford P. *Birthright: The Parents Choice*. London: BBC, 1985.

Inglis B, West R. *The Alternative Health Guide*. London: Michael Joseph, 1983.

Institute of Electrical Engineers. *Regulations for Electrical Installation*. 16th Edition. Hertfordshire: IEE, 1991.

Jenkins R, Murphy A. *Accountability, the Law and the Midwife*. London: South Bank University, 1993.

Johnson J, Odent M. *We are all Water Babies*. London: Dragons world, 1994.

Johnson P. Birth under water: To breathe or not to breathe. *B J Obstet Gynaecol* 1996, 102: 202-8.

Katz VL, McMurray R, Berry MJ, Cefalo RC. Fetal and uterine responses to immersion and exercise. *Obstet Gynecol* 1998, 72(2): 225-30.

Ketter D, Shelton BJ. Pregnant and physically fit too. *Am J Matern Child Nurs* 1984, 9(2): 120-2.

Khamis Y, Shaala S, Damarawy H, Toppozada M. Effect of heat on uterine contractions. *Int J Gynaecol Obstet* 1983, 21: 491-3.

Kitzinger S. *Freedom and Choice in Childbirth*. London: Penguin, 1987.

Klaus MH, Kennell J. *Parent Infant Bonding*. London: Mosby, 1982.

Knowsley J. Waterbirth mothers face test for HIV. *Sunday Telegraph*, 31 December 1995, p 9.

Leboyer F. *Birth Without Violence*. London: Mandarin, 1975.

Lenstrup C, Schantz A, Berget A, Feder E, Roseno H, Hertel J. Warm tub bath during delivery. *Acta Obstet Gynecol Scand* 1987, 66(8): 709-12.

Lichy R, Herzberg E. *The Waterbirth Handbook*. Bath: Gateway books, 1993.

Mason D, Edwards P. *Litigation: A risk management guide for midwives*. London: RCM, 1993.

McCandlish R, Renfrew M. Immersion in water during labour and/or birth. *Birth* 1993, 20(2): 79-85.

McCraw RK. Recent innovations in childbirth. *J Nurs Midwifery* 1989, 34(4): 206-10.

McNeese N. Waterbirth: The right to an informed choice. *Pre and Perinatal Psychology* 1988, 11(1): 16-7.

Melzack R, Wall PD. Pain mechanism: A new theory. *Science* 1965, 150 (3699): 971-9.

Milner I. Waterbabies. *Nursing Times 1988*, 84(1): 39-40.

Moore S. Pain relief in labour: An overview. *BJM* 1994, 2(10): 483-6.

Morris D. *Babywatching*. Kent: Mackays, 1991.

Napierala S. *Waterbirth: A midwife's perspective*. USA: Bergin and Garvey, 1994.

Neal MJ. *Medical Pharmacology at a Glance*. Oxford: Blackwell Scientific, 1987.

Newburgh LH. *Physiology of Heat Regulation*. London: Hafner, 1968.

NCT. *Labour and birth in water*. London: NCT, 1995.

Nicol G. *Finland*. London: Batsford, 1975.

Nyman L. *Water birth and the risk of infection. A case control study*. ICM Conference Proceedings, 1999.

O'Connell P. The waterbirth option. *Childbirth instructor* 1998 July/Aug: 28-31.

Odent M. (1981). The evolution of obstetrics in Pithiviers. *Birth and the Family* 1981, 8(1): 7-15.

Odent M. Birth under water. *Lancet* 1983, Dec 24/31: 1476-7.

Odent M. *Birth Reborn*. London: Fontana Collins, 1984.

Odent M. *Entering the World*. London: Marion Boyers, 1984.

Odent M. The fetus ejection reflex. *Birth* 1987, 14(2): 104-5.

Odent M. *Water and Sexuality*. London: Arkana, 1990.

Odent M. Can water immersion stop labour. *J Nurs Midwifery* 1997, 42(5): 414-6.

Oudshoorn C. Swimming class for pregnant women. Paper presented at ICM, 1990.

Pattison S. Taking the plunge. *NCT Journal* 1996, May: 66-9.

Pearce JC. *Magical Child*. London: Paladin Granada, 1977.

Power GG. Biology of temperature: The mammalian fetus. *Journal of Developmental Physiology* 1989, 12: 295–304.

Rawal J, Shah A, Stirk F. Birthing tub caused infection. *Nursing Times*, August 31st 1994, 90(35).

Ray S. *Ideal Birth*. Berkeley, USA: Celestial Arts, 1986.

RCM. *Normality in Midwifery*. London: RCM, 1997.

RCN. *Commissioning women-centred maternity care*. London: RCN, 1996.

RCN. *Manual handling assessments in hospital and the community*. London: RCN, 1996.

Ridgway G, Tedder RS. Birthing pools and infection control. *Lancet* 1996, 347(9007): 6.

Robinson J. A waterbirth death in Sweden. *AIMS Journal* 1994, 5(3): 7-8.

Riggs M. *The scented bath*. London: Robert Hale, 1991.

Robinson J. AIMS and the ethics of a clinical trial. *AIMS Journal* 1994, 6(4): 1-5.

Robinson J. Waterbirth: False hopes, false promises. *AIMS Journal* 1996, 8(3): 17-8.

Rosenthal M. Warm water immersion in labor and birth. *The Female Patient* 1991, 16: 35.

Rogers J, Wood J, McCandlish R, Ayers S, Truesdale A, Elbourne D. Active versus expectant management of third stage of labour: The Hinchingbrooke randomised controlled trial. *Lancet* 1998, 351: 693-9.

Rosser, J. Is waterbirth safe? *MIDIRS Midwifery Digest* 1994, 4(1).

Royal College of Midwives. *The use of water during birth*. Position paper No. 1. London: RCM, 1994.

Rush J, Burlock S, Lambert K, Loosley-Millman M, Hutchinson B, Enkin M. The effects of whirlpool baths in labour: A randomised controlled trial. *Birth* 1996, 23(3): 136-43.

Salariya EM, Easton PM, Cater JI. Duration of feeding after early invitation and frequent feeding. *Lancet 1978*, ii: 1141-3.

Sidenbladh E. *Waterbabies*. London: Adam and Charles Black, 1983.

Simkin P. Hydrotherapy. *Effective Care in Pregnancy and Childbirth* 1990, 2: 898-9.

Skinner AT, Thomson AM. *Duffields Exercise in Water*. London: Bailliere Tindall, 1986.

Stanway A. *Alternative Medicine*. London: McDonalds and James, 1979.

Star RB. *The Healing Power of Birth*. Texas: Star, 1986.

Street D. Waterbirths: Client choice versus legal implications. *Nursing Times* 1997, 93(45): 50-1.

Tiran D, Mack S. *Complementary Therapies for Pregnancy and Childbirth*. London: Bailliere Tindall, 1994.

UKCC. *Code of Professional Conduct*. London: UKCC, 1984.

UKCC. *Midwives Code of Practice*. London: UKCC, 1991.

UKCC. *Midwives Rules*. London: UKCC, 1991.

UKCC. *Midwives Rules*. London: UKCC, 1993.

UKCC. *Waterbirth: The current position*. London: UKCC, 1996.

UKCC. *Midwives rules and code of Practice*. London: UKCC, 1998.

University of Case Western Ohio. *University Obstetrics/Gynaecology Specialities Report*. Cleveland Ohio, USA: University Hospitals, 1992.

Verny T. *The Secret Life of the Unborn Child*. London: Sphere Books, 1987.

Wambach H. *Life Before Life*. London/New York: Bantam Books, 1979.

Weston CFM, O'Hare JP, Evans JM, Corrall RJM. Haemodynamic changes in man during immersion in water at different temperatures. *Clinical Science* 1987, 73: 613-16.

Zimmermann R, Huch A, Huch R. Waterbirth: Is it safe? *Journal of Perinatal Medicine* 1993, 21: 5-11.

Recommended Further Reading

Abidin MR, Becker DG, Dang MT, Edlich RF, Pavlovich LJ. Design of hydrotherapy exercise pools. *JBCR* 1987, Sept/Oct: 505-9.

Adamsons K. Thermal homeostasis in the Towell, ME fetus and newborn. *Anesthesiology* 1965, July-August: 531-47.

Burnard P, Chapman CM. *Professional and Ethical Issues in Nursing.* Chichester: Wiley and sons, 1988.

Chapman V. Waterbirths: Breakthrough or burden? *BJM* 1994, 2(1): 17-9.

Church LK. Waterbirth: One birthing centre's observations. *J Nurs Midwifery* 1989, 34(4): 165.

Deschenes L. L'hydrotherapie. *Nursing Quebec* 1990, 10(3).

Dimond B. *Legal Aspects of Nursing.* New York: Prentice Hall, 1990.

Dimond B. Waterbirths: The legal implications for midwives. *Modern Midwife* 1994, January: 12-13.

Dimond B. *Legal Aspects of Midwifery.* Manchester: Books for Midwives, 1994.

Elbourne DR. Active v conservative third-stage management. Pregnancy and Childbirth Module. *Cochrane Database.* Review 05353.Disk issue 1 1994.

Fernandes L. My water baby. *Baby magazine,* Oct 1998, 39-40.

Ford L, Garland D. An aquabirth concept. *Midwives Chronicle* 1989, 102: 232-34.

Garland D. *Professional Report: The Ohio Experience.* Maidstone Health Authority, 1989.

Garland D. *Professional Report: Waterbirth Clinical Visits.* Maidstone Health Authority, 1992.

Gillett GB, Watson JD, Langford RM. Ranitidine and single dose antacid therapy. *Anaesthesia* 1984, 39: 638-44.

Gillot de Vries, Wesel S, Busine A, Camus AM, Patesson R, Gillard C. Influence of a bath during labor on the experience of maternity. *Pre and Perinatal Psychology* 1987, 1(4): 297-302.

Ginesi L. Waterbirth. *NCT Annual* 1991, 106-7.

Gordon Y. Water birth: A personal view. *Maternal and Child Health* 1991, 168: 245-6.

Griscom C. *Ocean Born.* Munich: Wilheim Verlas, 1989.

Herzberg E. Waterbabies. *The Best of Health,* May 1986.

Hinchliff S, Montegue S. *Physiology for Nursing Practice.* London: Bailliere Tindall, 1991.

House of Commons Health Committee. *Maternity Services.* London: HMSO, 1992.

McCandlish R, Renfrew M. Immersion in water during labour and birth. *Birth* 1993, 20(2): 79-85.

Moir DD, Thorburn J. *Obstetrics, Anaesthesia and Analgesia.* London: Bailliere Tindall, 1986.

Odent M. Birth under water. *Lancet* 1983, Dec. 24-31: 1476-7.

Parkes R. Isabella's birthday. *Midwifery Matters* 1998, Issue 76. Spring: 13-5.

Petrikovsky BM, Schneider EP. Underwater birth. *The Female Patient* 1997, 22 (Feb): 29-36.

Pyne RH. *Professional Discipline in Nursing, Midwifery and Health Visiting.* London: Blackwell Scientific, 1992.

Rush J. (1992). Effect of warm whirlpool baths during labour. Cited: Chalmers, I. Oxford database. 1.2 Disk 8 No. 6382.

Schreuder C. Underwater births arise as a mainstream option. *Chicago Tribune,* Friday October 18th 1996, p 2a-2b.

MATERNAL/FETAL INTERDEPENDENCY

Maternal hormones

Adrenaline and noradrenaline affect all major systems

Secreted from Adrenal Medulla

	Adrenaline 80%	Noradrenaline 20%
Effects on nervous system	Wakefulness/emotions	Anxiety
Effects on cardiovascular system	Cardiac output Peripheral resistance Systolic blood pressure Diastolic blood pressure	Blood pressure Pallor Sweat Anxiety
Effects on respiratory system	Metabolic rate Energy utilisation Heat production Oxygen consumption	

Feedback via nerve impulses to hypothalamus. Increased adrenaline levels with hypothermia and hypoglycaemia.

Fetal awareness of internal and external factors

Alcohol	Drugs	Smoking
Maternal position	Infections	Diet
'Stress' hormones	Maternal fears	Anxiety
Uterine changes	Contractions	Intrauterine pressure

Protection

Placenta	Antibodies	'Own' hormones
Genetic makeup		

HYPERTHERMIA

In studies undertaken on pregnant ewes there is some evidence that maternal hyperthermia could have a profound effect on fetal temperature and heart rate (Cefalo *et al*, 1978). Heat application to the uterus whilst contracting appears to cause an accelerated local metabolic rate and arteriolar dilation (Khamis, 1983). With all these issues in mind it is worth reviewing the mechanism of temperature and effects of hyperthermia.

Mechanism of heat balance regulation

Heat regulation
Control via anterior hypothalamus – which protects against over heating/over cooling.

Long-term heat adjustments involve pituitary, thyroid and adrenal glands.

Hypothalamus
Anterior region:
• optic chiasma and anterior commissure, prevent overheating
• assists through vasodilation and sweating.

Posterior region:
• corpora mammillaria protects from cold
• assists through vasoconstriction and shivering.

There is an interplay between the two lobes.

Maintenance of core temperature at 37°C through peripheral thermo-ceptors in skin and the reflex that occurs at this level and hyporeceptors via circulating blood. (Bazett, cited in Newburgh,1968.)

Heat gain

- Metabolism – increased tissue metabolism occurs with exercise to 39°C – is affected by circulating thyroxine.

- External environment – increases core temperature if greater than ambient temperature.

- Hot foods and drinks cause a minimal raise in temperature.

- Hormones
  - some hormones cause a rise in temperature:
  - thyroxine – a little effect
  - adrenaline – in hot environments adrenaline is secreted into the blood stream; its function is to cause modifications to blood supply in favour to muscle (uterus), liberation of glucose which can be assimilated and an increase in heat production.
  - noradrenaline
  - progesterone – a little.

- Layers of adipose brown fat.
  (Newburgh, 1968)

Heat loss

Eighty-five per cent of heat loss occurs through conduction and convection.

- Conduction – little loss through cooler direct surface contact. Heat conducted from within the body to skin surface and out to any cooler surface.
- Convection – heat transfer is dependent upon physical transfer of a liquid or gas. Streams of air rise from a warm surface. Increased air circulation causes increased convection.
- Radiation – is the exchange of thermal energy between objects, through a process which depends only upon the temperature and the nature of the surfaces of the radiating objects. Heat passes through the skin to other objects in its path.
- Evaporation – this causes physiological control of water evaporation from the body via the skin and lungs. If the skin is moist then there

is an increased evaporation. Skin to air exchange occurs a few millimetres from skin surface, thus if there is not an ambient temperature, with stagnant air this energy transfer may be reduced.

Water loss also occurs into the environment through sweating.

Minimal heat loss also occurs through urine/faeces and respiratory tract.

Effects of hydrotherapy and hyperthermia

Normal heat

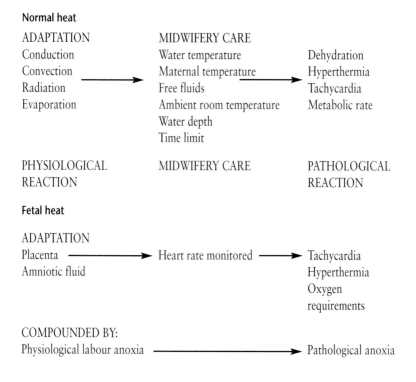

ADAPTATION
Conduction
Convection
Radiation
Evaporation

MIDWIFERY CARE
Water temperature
Maternal temperature
Free fluids
Ambient room temperature
Water depth
Time limit

Dehydration
Hyperthermia
Tachycardia
Metabolic rate

PHYSIOLOGICAL
REACTION

MIDWIFERY CARE

PATHOLOGICAL
REACTION

Fetal heat

ADAPTATION
Placenta
Amniotic fluid

Heart rate monitored

Tachycardia
Hyperthermia
Oxygen
requirements

COMPOUNDED BY:
Physiological labour anoxia

Pathological anoxia

WATERBIRTH PARENTS EVENING
Suggested format

- Introductions

- Why choose water?
  Theory and practice
  World-wide perspective

- Will tubs be available?
  Home or hospital use?

- Will midwives be available?
  (What support and education do they receive?)

- Your partner's role

- Guidelines for practice

- Advantages or not? What is the latest evidence?

- Caring for you and your baby. Monitoring fluids/temperatures

- Video, and disussion of
  Partner's role
  Third stage management
  Newborn physiology

- Unit statistics – audit forms

- Your questions answered

- Tour of waterbirthing rooms

- Resources and contacts

HOME WATERBIRTH FOLLOW-UP LETTER

Dear ...

Thank you for inviting me to your home to discuss the planning of your home waterbirth.

May I take this opportunity to confirm that we discussed:

– Calling of the community midwife and her back up system for a second midwife.

– The education and support given to staff to ensure they are able to offer you a home waterbirth.

– Ambulance response times (… minutes) and reasons for transfer to hospital.

– Equipment carried by the midwife – including that required for homebirth, and the extras required for waterbirth (underwater doppler, sieve, water thermometer, plastic mirror, flotation aids).

– Watertub – weight of the structure and nature of the floor. Positioning of the tub, access to water. Home insurance (we suggest you check your home insurance policy) and use of electrical equipment near to water. We suggest that you undertake a 'dry' run and speak to the midwife if you have any problems.

– May I confirm that it is your partner's responsibility to ensure the tub is set up and kept filled. The water tank will probably hold 40-60 gallons. As several refills may be necessary, I would suggest that you fill the tub early in labour, and cover with the thermal cover provided.

– If children or pets are in the home, please be careful when the tub is full. If children are to be present during labour, ensure that a separate birth companion is available for them.

– We discussed when to enter the water (in established labour, as it can slow or stop non-established labour).

In an emergency you will be asked to leave the water.

– Third stage options – in or out of water.

Thank you again for your time. If I can assist in any way, please do not hesitate to contact me.

Yours Sincerely

cc Mother's file/Community midwife.

GUIDELINES FOR PROTECTING YOUR BACK

Waterbirths and the need to adopt alternative positions for delivery may pose new challenges for midwives, with regard to health and safety.

Because there is a need to have deep, wide tubs, midwives may find that they need to review several issues prior to using them.

- Review your own professional responsibility towards health and safety. When did you last attend a training session?

- Review current practice on positions adopted when assisting mothers to breastfeed or deliver in alternative positions.

- Risk assessment should be undertaken with senior midwifery staff and a Health and Safety representative. It is not always possible to eradicate risk. However, it is important that it is reduced to the lowest possible level.

- Midwives should take every opportunity to undertake a 'dry' run, at home or hospital. Where will you sit, kneel? Is extra equipment required (for example, stools, cushions or beanbags)? All options and positions should be explored.

- Hoists and lifting equipment may be available when tubs are particularly deep.

- Responsibility at home should be discussed with parents.

- If you have a history of back or spinal problems you should inform your Supervisor of Midwives and seek health advice and support from the Occupational Health Department.

Reference
Manual handling assessments in hospital and the community. RCN, 1996.

USEFUL ADDRESSES

British Paediatric Surveillance Unit
30 Guildford Street,
London WC1N 1EH
Tel: 0207 242 9789

HNE Diagnostics
35 Portanmoor Road,
Cardiff CF2 2HB
(underwater monitor)

MIDIRS
9 Elmdale Road, Clifton,
Bristol BS8 1SL
Tel: 0117 925 1791

MIRIAD
University of Leeds,
24 Hyde Terrace, Leeds LS2 9LN
Tel: 0113 233 6888

Oxford Sonicaid
1 Kimber Road, Abingdon, Oxon
OX14 1BZ
(underwater monitor)

Silverlea Textiles
27 Totnes Road, Newton Abbot,
Devon TQ12 1LU
(patient lifting sling)

WATERBIRTH TUB COMPANIES

Active Birth Centre
Bickerton House,
25 Bickerton Road,
London N19 5JT
Tel: 0207 482 5554

Aqua Babies
20 Harrison Close, Broadhinton,
Twyford, Reading RG10 OLL

Birth Rites
3 Gage Road, Forest Row,
East Sussex RH18 5HL
Tel: 01342 826581

Birthworks
4E Brent Mill Trading Estate,
South Brent, Devon TQ10 9YT

Centromed
Unit 5, Stafford Close,
Fairwood Industrial Park, Ashford,
Kent TN23 2TT

Glass Fibre Mouldings
Unit 5, The Colt Works,
Pluckley Road, Bethersden, Kent

**Global Maternal/
Child Health Association**
PO Box 1400, Wilsonville,
Oregon 97070, USA

Splash down
17 Wellington Terrace,
Harrow-on-the-Hill, Middlesex
Tel: 0208 422 9308

AQUAROBIC AQUANATAL COURSES

Aquarobics Ltd
356 Dover House Road,
London SW15 5BL
Tel: 0208 788 2471

Aquarobics
148 White Hart Lane,
London SW13 OJP
Tel: 0208 878 9868

WATERBIRTHS WORLDWIDE

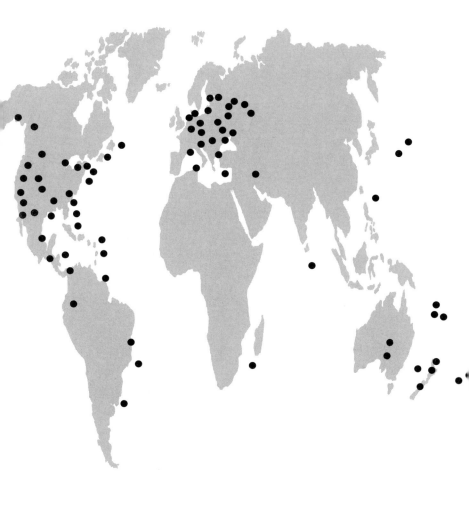

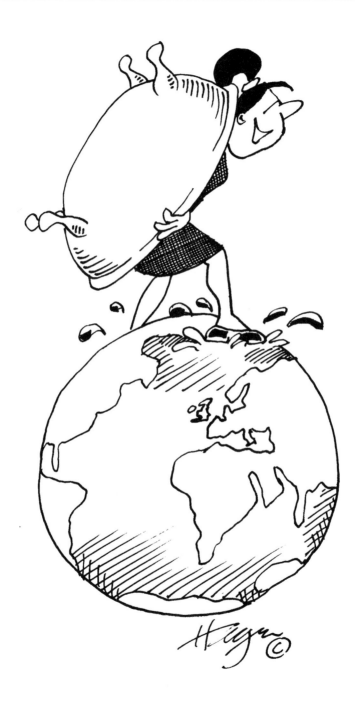

Index

entering/leaving, 42–3
hiring of, 41–2, 45
infection control, 48–9, 92–3, 126
setting up at home, 45–6
water contamination, 107–8

Ultrasound, 76

Vicarious liability, 6

Water:
benefits of in pain relief, 72–4
contamination, 107–8
spillage, 49
temperature, 66–7

therapeutic value of, 9–14
Waterbirth, 13–15, 18–24
America, 27–32
at home, 41–2
Europe, 32–7
fetal perspective on, 79–82
guidelines, 51–3
quiz, 119–20
reasons for, 65
room design, 40–1
ten-point plan, 53–4
Waterbirth International (WBI), 21, 27
Winterton Report, 14, 18, 38, 79
Working together, 3

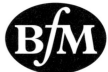
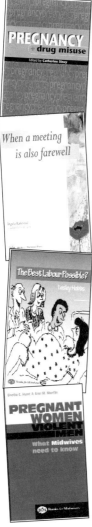